GRAMMAR AND PUNCTUATION

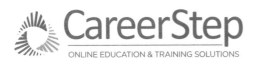

ONLINE EDUCATION & TRAINING SOLUTIONS

Career Step, LLC
Phone: 801.489.9393
Toll-Free: 800.246.7837
Fax: 801.491.6645
careerstep.com

This text companion contains a snapshot of the online program content converted to a printed format. Please note that the online training program is constantly changing and improving and is always the source of the most up-to-date information.

Product Number: HG-PR-11-002
Generation Date: September 23, 2013

TABLE OF CONTENTS

UNIT 1

Introduction

INTRODUCTION TO GRAMMAR AND PUNCTUATION

Learning Objective

This module is a refresher of basic English grammar and punctuation rules. Upon completion, the student will be able to recognize and identify proper usage, language, and punctuation.

One very important skill required for producing quality medical reports is a working knowledge of English grammar. You need to know how to construct a proper sentence with the correct employment of usage, capitalization, and punctuation. Thus, it is essential that you be familiar and comfortable with the basic rules of English grammar.

As a medical transcription editor, the responsibility of creating an accurate document lies with you. Generally speaking, at the worst, you will be permitted a maximum of two errors per page. This includes punctuation, grammar, spelling, and formatting. Furthermore, you should know that although sometimes doctors will dictate punctuation in their reports, they will often dictate it incorrectly, and *you* are responsible for seeing that it is corrected.

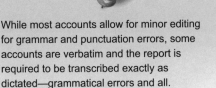

While most accounts allow for minor editing for grammar and punctuation errors, some accounts are verbatim and the report is required to be transcribed exactly as dictated—grammatical errors and all.

This module on grammar is designed to be a refresher course. You studied English in school, and this is intended as a review of some of those rules. Unlike English in school, however, you will rarely (if ever) be required to write or to come up with your own original sentences and paragraphs. You will only be editing and clarifying the work of the dictating physicians. This is an important thing to keep in mind as you work through these exercises.

As is the case throughout the program, you will be tested at the end of each unit. Your scores should never be less than 85% before going on to other units.

UNIT 2

Parts of Speech

PARTS OF SPEECH – INTRODUCTION

Unless you are an English teacher or you learned English as a second language, you probably give little thought to the types and functions of the words you use when you speak. We internalize the rules of the English language when we learn to speak. Then, through repetitive practice we learn to build sentences correctly (usually). As a medical transcription editor, however, an "organic" knowledge of the English language is not enough. Because you are using the doctor's spoken words to create a detailed legal document, accuracy is paramount. To be accurate, you must know the basics as well as the advanced rules governing the language. So in our effort to review and re-acquaint you with the rules of grammar and punctuation, we will start with the basics: the parts of speech.

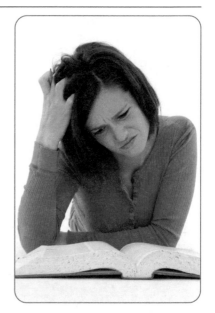

You probably have not thought about the parts of speech since your teacher made you diagram sentences and you wondered why she was torturing you in such a way. While that painful method was effective for some, we are going to forgo diagramming and focus on the **roles** the parts of speech play in building good sentences.

While anyone can memorize the definitions of the parts of speech (there are only 8 of them), knowing the definitions does not do any good unless you can understand the function of the parts of speech within a sentence. You may be getting a hint of that torturous feeling again, but relax… it won't be that bad. It is imperative that you understand the function of individual words because they are the basic building blocks of our complex language. Good words make good phrases and clauses, which make good sentences, which make good paragraphs, which make perfect reports… and that, after all, is your goal!

PARTS OF SPEECH

Without further ado, let's re-introduce you to the eight parts of speech:

Noun: Word used to name a person, place, thing, or idea.

Pronoun: Word used in place of a noun.

Adjective: Word used to modify a noun or a pronoun.

Verb: Word that expresses action or shows a state of being.

Adverb: Word used to modify a verb, adjective, or other adverb.

Preposition: Word that shows the relation of a noun to another word in the sentence.

Conjunction: Word that joins other words/groups of words.

Interjection: Word that adds emotion to a sentence (Wow!). Since these are almost never used in medical reports, we will not spend time on interjections.

The way each part of speech behaves in a sentence and its interaction with the other words in the sentence is what you must understand to make clear, correct sentences. Many of the words in our language can be more than one part of speech. You must know the word's **role** in the sentence to understand what part of speech it is in that particular instance.

The patient's mother said the child would **scream** every time she bent her finger.
The patient's mother said she heard a **scream** coming from her daughter's room.

*In the first sentence, **scream** is an action—a verb.*
*In the second sentence, **scream** is a thing—a noun.*

Only by understanding the function of the word and those surrounding it would you be able to know what part of speech the word is.

The nice thing about this unit is that you are familiar with the information because you build sentences every time you speak or write. All we are doing is naming and explaining that which you already know.

NOUNS AND PRONOUNS

Nouns are words that represent people, places, things, or ideas.

People: brother, minister, wife, Nancy Reagan, teacher, Arnold Palmer

Place: school, Earth, store, New Mexico, home

Thing: table, chicken, leg, Washington Monument, chewing gum, Toyota truck

Idea: love, honor, fear, anger, hatred

Nouns that are capitalized are called **proper nouns**. They point out specific people, places, or things. Nouns that are not capitalized are called **common nouns**.

Nouns can come anywhere in a sentence—the beginning, middle, or end.

My dog is going to the kennel in late February.
***February** is a proper noun. **Dog** and **kennel** are common nouns.*

I miss Florida because we would get sunshine throughout the winter.
***Florida** is a proper noun. **Sunshine** and **winter** are common nouns.*

She said her jealousy for Abbey started as a little thing and grew into a monster.
***Abbey** is a proper noun. **Jealousy**, **thing**, and **monster** are common nouns.*

Remember the idea of looking at a word's **function** in the sentence rather than just the definition of the particular part of speech. A word that is a noun can also be used to describe another noun. The word is then considered an adjective because of its **function** in the sentence.

The patient has a history of colon cancer.

*Although **colon** is a noun (a thing), in this case it is modifying the word **cancer**. It would be considered an adjective in this sentence.*

She complains of joint pain in her left elbow.

Again, **joint** is usually a noun. In this case, it modifies the word **pain**, so it is considered an adjective.

A **pronoun** is a word that takes the place of a noun. We use pronouns because our sentences would become long, redundant, and confusing if we only used nouns.

Janet's daughter brought Janet's daughter's lunch to Janet's daughter's first day of kindergarten.

Help! We need pronouns!

Janet's daughter brought her lunch to her first day of kindergarten.

Whew. Much better.

There are many types of pronouns, but all of them have one thing in common: they replace a noun. While you will not be expected to identify each of the different types of pronouns, they will be explained here so you can see the functions they have within different sentences.

Who ate mine?

Who *is an interrogative pronoun (pronoun used to ask a question). It takes the place of the person who ate the food. The other interrogative pronouns are* **which, what**, *and* **whom**.

Mine *is a possessive pronoun that takes the place of the speaker and shows his/her ownership of the food (before someone ate it, of course). The other possessive pronouns are* **yours, hers, his, its, ours, whose**, *and* **theirs**. *If they precede a noun, they are* **my, your, her, his, their, its, our, whose**.

This is too heavy for me.

This *takes the place of whatever the thing is that is heavy. It is a demonstrative pronoun, which points to a thing or person. The other demonstrative pronouns are* **that, these**, *and* **those**.

Me *is a personal pronoun—the most common kind. It takes the place of a person. The other personal pronouns are* **I, you, he, she, it, we, they, me, her, him, us, them**. *Of course, they change forms depending upon the number and gender of the people they replace.*

Everything John found was returned to the person who lost it.

Everything *takes place of all of the items John found. This is called an indefinite pronoun because it replaces things/people that are not specific. Some other indefinite pronouns are* **everyone, anyone, someone, any, all, few, many, none, nobody, somebody**.

Who *is a relative pronoun in this case. A relative pronoun relates to a noun that precedes it in the sentence. It connects a dependent clause to the noun that it relates to. In this sentence* **who** *relates to* **person** *(and connects* **who lost it** *to the person). These are probably the most difficult pronouns to identify. The other relative pronouns are* **whoever, which, that, and whom**.

ADJECTIVES

If you have ever known someone who loves to work on cars, you may have seen him modify the automobile in some way. Perhaps he added a new exhaust system or changed the stereo or even painted the body of the car… all of those are examples of **modifying** a car. Similarly, the job of an adjective is to **modify** a noun or pronoun. To modify a noun, an **adjective** can describe the noun, add more information about it, or quantify it. An adjective will answer one of the following three questions about the noun it modifies:

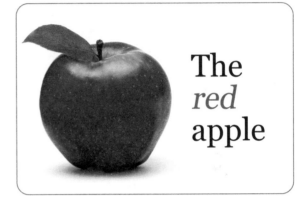

The
red
apple

1. Which one?
2. What kind?
3. How many?

The patient was referred for radiation therapy.

*The adjective **radiation** modifies the noun **therapy** by telling **what kind** of therapy.*

She presented with two lesions on her cheek.

*The adjective **two** modifies the noun **lesion** by telling **how many** lesions.*

We asked her to return to this clinic on Monday.

*The adjective **this** modifies the noun **clinic** by telling **which clinic**.*

*Note—Remember the word **this** was also a pronoun when used by itself in a sentence. It is an adjective when it precedes a noun because it modifies the noun. It's all about the **function** of the word!*

Possessive pronouns can also be used as adjectives. When they modify a noun or pronoun, they are functioning as an adjective rather than a pronoun.

She was asked to raise her arm.

*Since the word **her** is modifying the noun **arm** by telling **which arm**, it is considered an adjective.*

Remember the interrogative pronouns (those that ask a question)? They can also function as adjectives. Just look at the function of the word in the sentence.

Which medications were prescribed?

*The word **which** modifies the noun **medications** by telling (or in this case, asking) which medication.*

I. **MULTIPLE CHOICE.**
The following sentences have some nouns, pronouns, and adjectives which are in orange. Choose the correct part of speech for each orange word. If it is an adjective, enter the noun that it modifies in the box provided.

She describes the pain as sharp pain located in the right trochanteric region.

1. She
   - ○ noun
   - ⊘ pronoun
   - ○ adjective. What noun does it modify? _____

2. sharp
   - ○ noun
   - ○ pronoun
   - ⊘ adjective. What noun does it modify? _pain_

3. right
   - ○ noun
   - ○ pronoun
   - ⊘ adjective. What noun does it modify? _trochanteric_

4. trochanteric
   - ○ noun
   - ○ pronoun
   - ⊘ adjective. What noun does it modify? _region_

Extremities are without clubbing*, cyanosis, or edema.

"Clubbing"—though the "ing" marks it as a verbal form, it functions as a noun. Such a noun is called a gerund. You don't have to remember that!

5. Extremities
   - ⊘ noun
   - ○ pronoun
   - ○ adjective. What noun does it modify? _____

6. clubbing
   - ⊘ noun
   - ○ pronoun
   - ○ adjective. What noun does it modify? _____

7. cyanosis
   - ⊘ noun
   - ○ pronoun
   - ○ adjective. What noun does it modify? _____

8. edema
   - ⊘ noun
   - ○ pronoun
   - ○ adjective. What noun does it modify? _____

The patient is a black female who awoke with severe retrosternal chest pain.

9. who
   - ○ noun
   - ⊘ pronoun
   - ○ adjective. What noun does it modify? _____

10. severe
    - ○ noun
    - ○ pronoun
    - ⊘ adjective. What noun does it modify? _pain_____

11. pain
    - ⊘ noun
    - ○ pronoun
    - ○ adjective. What noun does it modify? _____

The medial and lateral gutters revealed a small amount of debris.

12. medial
    - ○ noun
    - ○ pronoun
    - ⊘ adjective. What noun does it modify? _medial_____

13. lateral
    - ○ noun
    - ○ pronoun
    - ⊘ adjective. What noun does it modify? _lateral_____

14. debris
- ⊘ noun
- ◯ pronoun
- ◯ adjective. What noun does it modify? _____

The lateral compartment revealed grade II changes of the lateral tibial plateau.

15. lateral
- ◯ noun
- ◯ pronoun
- ⊘ adjective. What noun does it modify? *Compartment*

16. compartment
- ⊘ noun
- ◯ pronoun
- ◯ adjective. What noun does it modify? _____

17. tibial
- ◯ noun
- ◯ pronoun
- ⊘ adjective. What noun does it modify? *Plateau*

18. plateau
- ⊘ noun
- ◯ pronoun
- ◯ adjective. What noun does it modify? _____

The patient tolerated the procedure well and was transferred from the operating room to the recovery room without incident.

19. patient
- ⊘ noun
- ◯ pronoun
- ◯ adjective. What noun does it modify? _____

20. operating
- ◯ noun
- ◯ pronoun
- ⊘ adjective. What noun does it modify? *room*

21. incident
- ⊘ noun
- ◯ pronoun
- ◯ adjective. What noun does it modify? _____

Hemostasis was maintained using the Bovie cautery.

22. Hemostasis
- ⊘ noun
- ◯ pronoun
- ◯ adjective. What noun does it modify? _____

23. Bovie
- ◯ noun
- ◯ pronoun
- ⊘ adjective. What noun does it modify? ___Cautery___

24. cautery
- ⊘ noun
- ◯ pronoun
- ◯ adjective. What noun does it modify? _____

VERBS

The verb is the most important part of speech because a sentence cannot exist without a verb. It is the only part of speech that is essential to a sentence… you can have a sentence without a noun or an adjective or a pronoun, but you cannot have a sentence without a verb. Why not? Simply put, the verb acts like the engine of a car—it makes the sentence "go." A **verb** gives action to or expresses the state of being of the thing (noun or pronoun) the sentence is about.

> The patient fell from her porch several days ago.
>
> *The word **fell** gives action to the noun **patient**. Without the verb, this would not be a sentence.*
>
> He stretches every morning.
>
> *The verb **stretches** gives action to the pronoun **he**.*

In addition to showing action, verbs can show a state of being. The verbs that show state of being are called **linking verbs**. They link the noun or pronoun to another word (usually an adjective or another noun).

The patient is a cashier.

*The verb **is** links the noun **patient** to the noun **cashier**, showing us the state of the patient.*

She seems content with the current program.

*The verb **seems** links the pronoun **she** to the adjective **content**, showing us the state of this female.*

*The most common linking verbs are the verbs of being: **be, been, being, is, am, are, was, were**.*

*There are other verbs that are commonly used as linking verbs: **become, seem, appear, look, feel.***

Occasionally, a proper noun is genericized and morphed into a verb by public use (or overuse). For example, we often *xerox* things (make copies). If you aren't sure if you should cap the word *Xerox* when used as a verb, you can *google* it (use the Google search engine to find information on the World Wide Web). You might also *tivo* your favorite TV show because you are going out of town. When we verbify a proper noun, we typically drop the capitalization, but that is not a steadfast rule. For example, *Google* is in some English dictionaries capped as both a proper noun and a verb.

Verbs can change forms depending upon the number of the nouns or pronouns that they are giving action to or linking.

One man goes to the emergency room.

But

Two men go to the emergency room.

We will cover this in detail in a future unit on agreement. But verbs can also change form depending upon tense. Many times, it will take a compound verb to accurately express tense. A **compound verb** is simply a main verb plus one or more helping verbs.

The patient will be going to Radiology in the near future.

***Going** is the main verb, and the helping verbs **will** and **be** express a specific tense (in this case the simple future tense).*

They were skiing when the accident occurred.

***Skiing** is the main verb and **were** is the helping verb. Combined they give us a specific tense (in this case the past progressive tense).*

She will not undergo the procedure at this time.

Sometimes the compound verb is split by an adverb (not, never, finally, etc.) They are NOT part of the verb.

ADVERBS

An adverb is used commonly to modify an adjective, another adverb, or a verb. If modifying a verb, it can tell **how**, **when**, **where**, or **to what extent** (how often or how much) the action is done.

He drives carefully. (how)
He drives early. (when)
He can almost drive. (to what extent, how much)
He drives everywhere. (where)

Adverbs such as *actually, indeed, truly,* and *really* that modify verbs can also be used for emphasis.

She can really sing.
He is indeed sick.

An adverb can also modify an adjective.

He is a really good driver.*
The patient was desperately afraid of facing surgery.
It was an abnormally high fever.

*__Really__ modifies the adjective **good**, as in "really good," not the noun "driver" (really driver?). If it were modifying the verb in this sentence, it would have to read, "He really is a good driver."*

An adverb can also modify another adverb.

He performed very well.

Very modifies **well**, which is an adverb because it modifies the verb **performed**: he performed well.

Occasionally a word can function as either a noun or an adverb.

He was sick yesterday. (adverb)
She will be discharged tomorrow. (adverb)
I think I will go today. (adverb)
Today is the first day of the rest of your life. (noun)
Yesterday was a lousy day. (noun)
Tomorrow will be worse. (noun)

In the following sentences, the adverb is highlighted and an arrow points to the word or words it modifies.

1. The patient was **assessed** clinically with pyelonephritis.

2. The patient **improved** rapidly after diuresis.

3. These symptoms **worsened** progressively over the next several days.

4. The sputum culture ultimately **grew** out normal flora.

5. He was initially **treated** with oxygen, requiring four liters to keep his saturations above 90%.

6. The lung sounds gradually **improved**.

7. He was essentially **asymptomatic**.

8. She **did** well postoperatively until the morning of admission.

9. He usually can **walk** and **exercise** and is quite vigorous.

10. His condition quickly **deteriorated**.

ADVERBS IN ACTION

The adverbs in the following examples function to specify time, place, intensity, and position.

We often visit our neighbor in the nursing home.
He rarely recognizes us.
Put it right there.
Here comes the nurse with the painkillers.
However you beg, the doctor will not give you any more morphine.
The tumor was first discovered three years ago.
It has never been treated with chemotherapy.
He always has a reaction to penicillin.

The patient had pain in the shoulders bilaterally.
Unfortunately, he left against medical advice before the treatment was complete.

I. MULTIPLE CHOICE.
For each sentence choose the word that is an adverb.

1. We discontinued the medicine immediately.
   - ◯ We
   - ◯ discontinued
   - ◯ medicine
   - ◯ immediately

2. The patient spoke normally.
   - ◯ The
   - ◯ patient
   - ◯ spoke
   - ◯ normally

3. The gait is somewhat hesitant.
   - ◯ gait
   - ◯ is
   - ◯ somewhat
   - ◯ hesitant

4. The area was unusually discolored.
   - ◯ area
   - ◯ was
   - ◯ unusually
   - ◯ discolored

5. She comes in for a checkup yearly.
   - ◯ comes
   - ◯ for
   - ◯ checkup
   - ◯ yearly

II. FILL IN THE BLANK.

Each sentence below has an adverb highlighted. Enter into the blank which word or words the adverb modifies.

1. I instructed the patient to return tomorrow.

   tomorrow modifies which word: _____

2. The patient was advised to return to the clinic immediately for any redness or swelling.

   immediately modifies which word: _____

3. The patient had definitely suffered a myocardial infarction.

   definitely modifies which word: _____

4. Pain and swelling progressed rapidly.

   rapidly modifies which word: _____

5. The subcutaneous tissues were copiously irrigated, and a few small bleeders were cauterized.

   copiously modifies which word: _____

6. He grossly exaggerated the severity of his pain.

   grossly modifies which word: _____

REVIEW: PARTS OF SPEECH

I. MULTIPLE CHOICE.
Choose the part of speech for each numbered word. (Pay attention to each word's function.) In the case of adjectives, enter the word(s) that they modify in the space beside the choice "adjective." For greater accuracy in scoring, be sure to type the words exactly as they appear, without extra spaces, and with no following or preceding punctuation.

This six-month-old female[1] presents[2] with a one-week[3] history of cough[4] and cold[5]. Over the past two days, the patient has had increasing[6] cough and respiratory problems. The mom noted[7] apneic[8] episodes while the baby was sleeping[9] and cyanosis[10] while she was crying.[11] The mom[12] noticed a scattered[13] red rash[14] on the patient's body. The mom currently[15] is giving[16] nebulizers at home two to three times per day. The patient[17] was[18] previously[19] being treated[20] with Reglan[21], but mom stopped[22] it[23] because she[24] did not think it was helping. The patient has been voiding normally.[25]

1. female
   - ◯ noun
   - ◯ pronoun
   - ◯ adjective. What noun does it modify? _____
   - ◯ verb
   - ◯ adverb

2. presents
   - ◯ noun
   - ◯ pronoun
   - ◯ adjective. What noun does it modify? _____
   - ◯ verb
   - ◯ adverb

3. one-week
   - ◯ noun
   - ◯ pronoun
   - ◯ adjective. What noun does it modify? _____
   - ◯ verb
   - ◯ adverb

4. cough
   - ◯ noun
   - ◯ pronoun
   - ◯ adjective. What noun does it modify? _____
   - ◯ verb
   - ◯ adverb

5. cold
   - ◯ noun
   - ◯ pronoun
   - ◯ adjective. What noun does it modify? _____
   - ◯ verb
   - ◯ adverb

6. increasing
   - ◯ noun
   - ◯ pronoun
   - ◯ adjective. What noun does it modify? _____
   - ◯ verb
   - ◯ adverb

7. noted
   - ○ noun
   - ○ pronoun
   - ○ adjective. What noun does it modify? _____
   - ○ verb
   - ○ adverb

8. apneic
   - ○ noun
   - ○ pronoun
   - ○ adjective. What noun does it modify? _____
   - ○ verb
   - ○ adverb

9. was sleeping
   - ○ noun
   - ○ pronoun
   - ○ adjective. What noun does it modify? _____
   - ○ verb
   - ○ adverb

10. cyanosis
   - ○ noun
   - ○ pronoun
   - ○ adjective. What noun does it modify? _____
   - ○ verb
   - ○ adverb

11. was crying
   - ○ noun
   - ○ pronoun
   - ○ adjective. What noun does it modify? _____
   - ○ verb
   - ○ adverb

12. mom
   - ○ noun
   - ○ pronoun
   - ○ adjective. What noun does it modify? _____
   - ○ verb
   - ○ adverb

13. scattered
- ⭘ noun
- ⭘ pronoun
- ⭘ adjective. What noun does it modify? _____
- ⭘ verb
- ⭘ adverb

14. rash
- ⭘ noun
- ⭘ pronoun
- ⭘ adjective. What noun does it modify? _____
- ⭘ verb
- ⭘ adverb

15. currently
- ⭘ noun
- ⭘ pronoun
- ⭘ adjective. What noun does it modify? _____
- ⭘ verb
- ⭘ adverb

16. is giving
- ⭘ noun
- ⭘ pronoun
- ⭘ adjective. What noun does it modify? _____
- ⭘ verb
- ⭘ adverb

17. patient
- ⭘ noun
- ⭘ pronoun
- ⭘ adjective. What noun does it modify? _____
- ⭘ verb
- ⭘ adverb

18. was
- ⭘ noun
- ⭘ pronoun
- ⭘ adjective. What noun does it modify? _____
- ⭘ verb
- ⭘ adverb

19. previously
   ◯ noun
   ◯ pronoun
   ◯ adjective. What noun does it modify? _____
   ◯ verb
   ◯ adverb

20. being treated
   ◯ noun
   ◯ pronoun
   ◯ adjective. What noun does it modify? _____
   ◯ verb
   ◯ adverb

21. Reglan
   ◯ noun
   ◯ pronoun
   ◯ adjective. What noun does it modify? _____
   ◯ verb
   ◯ adverb

22. stopped
   ◯ noun
   ◯ pronoun
   ◯ adjective. What noun does it modify? _____
   ◯ verb
   ◯ adverb

23. it
   ◯ noun
   ◯ pronoun
   ◯ adjective. What noun does it modify? _____
   ◯ verb
   ◯ adverb

24. she
   ○ noun
   ○ pronoun
   ○ adjective. What noun does it modify? _____
   ○ verb
   ○ adverb

25. normally
   ○ noun
   ○ pronoun
   ○ adjective. What noun does it modify? _____
   ○ verb
   ○ adverb

PREPOSITIONS

Prepositions are words that link a noun or pronoun to other words in a sentence. Prepositions come in phrases (conveniently called prepositional phrases) that act as one unit. That is important enough to reiterate: prepositional phrases act as a single unit. A prepositional phrase is made up of the preposition, the noun or pronoun that it is relating to (called the object of the preposition), and any adjectives or adverbs that may fall in between the two.

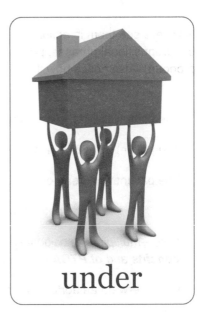

under

The wound on his scalp was cleaned.

On his scalp is the prepositional phrase. On is the preposition. Prepositional phrases always start with the preposition. Scalp is the object of the preposition. Prepositional phrases always end in the noun or pronoun that is the object of the preposition.

Prepositions show a spatial, time, or logical relationship between the object of the preposition and the rest of the sentence. In the example above, *on his scalp* shows the wound in terms of space—*where* in space is the wound? On his scalp. The most common prepositions are as follows:

aboard	between	past
about	beyond	since
above	but	through
across	by	throughout
after	down	to
against	during	toward
along	except	under
amid	for	underneath
among	from	until
around	in	unto
at	into	up
before	like	upon
behind	of	with
below	off	within
beneath	on	without
beside	over	

So any of these prepositions can be made into prepositional phrases by adding a noun after them and an adjective(s) or adverb(s) between them.

> aboard the boat
> between the pages
> since her last appointment
> from the injury

Now let's see them in action. The following sentences all contain prepositional phrases. Notice the pattern of the prepositional phrases: preposition → adjectives or adverbs (optional) → object of the preposition (noun or pronoun). Also notice how they act as a single unit (like a single part of speech).

> The contusion on her arm seems to be healing at this time.
>
> The patient is a 63-year-old white female with no previous cardiac history.
>
> The patient was treated with thrombolytic therapy.
>
> After the exam, the patient was advised of the risks and benefits of PTCA.
>
> *Note—multiple prepositional phrases often come back to back, like the phrases **of the risks and benefits** and **of PTCA** in this sentence.*
>
> He underwent an aortobifemoral bypass in 1985.
>
> At that time, the patient had URI symptoms and was treated with antibiotics.
>
> A second port was made along the 6th intercostal space.
>
> The patient was taken to the recovery room in good condition.
>
> *Note—Again, this sentence contains two prepositional phrases back to back.*

Test yourself on these sentences. Identify the prepositional phrases in the following sentences

1. The patient will now undergo a thoracoscopic lung biopsy of the left lung.
2. Her potassium was 2.8 on admission.
3. For that reason, nursing home placement procedures will be done by the hospital social worker.
4. The patient was admitted for a workup of his suspected atherosclerotic peripheral vascular disease.
5. Attention was turned to the descending portion of the colon which was released on its antimesentery border by electrocautery along the white line of Toldt.

I. **TRUE/FALSE.**
If the orange words highlighted are a prepositional phrase, mark True. If they are not, mark False.

1. The splenic flexure was carefully reduced using sharp and electrocautery technique.
   ○ true
   ○ false

2. This is a 6-year-old male who took an unknown amount of Dilantin at approximately 9:30 on the morning of admission.
   ○ true
   ○ false

3. Normally, this patient walks on his toes and does not talk a lot.
   ○ true
   ○ false

4. He lives with his 2 siblings and his parents.
   ○ true
   ○ false

5. He was born by normal spontaneous vaginal delivery with Apgars of 9 and 10.
   ○ true
   ○ false

6. The abdomen was prepped and draped in the usual sterile fashion.
   ○ true
   ○ false

7. He was then awakened from general endotracheal anesthesia, extubated, and returned to the recovery room.
   ○ true
   ○ false

8. He has been on omeprazole for 2 weeks prior to current visit, although it was prescribed 1 month ago.
   ○ true
   ○ false

9. He has a history of undocumented uric acid stones with urinary retention and urinary tract infection in 1999.
   ○ true
   ○ false

10. With dissection, the cricopharyngeus muscle became evident, as did the moderately large esophageal diverticulum arising just superior to the cricopharyngeus muscle.
    ○ true
    ○ false

CONJUNCTIONS

Conjunctions are words that join words, phrases, or clauses. The most common type of conjunction is the coordinating conjunction. A **coordinating conjunction** joins two parts of a sentence that are equal in importance. I was taught to remember FANBOYS to help recall the coordinating conjunctions: F=For, A=And, N=Nor, B=But, O=Or, Y=Yet, S=So.

> The patient's posture and gait are normal.
> *The conjunction **and** joins the nouns **posture** and **gait**. The two words have equal roles in the sentence.*
>
> The patient will return or call if things worsen.
> *The conjunction **or** joins the verbs **return** and **call**.*
>
> She appeared comfortable, but I wished to keep her for observation.
> *The conjunction **but** joins the two independent clauses (sentences).*

Correlative conjunctions are very similar to coordinating conjunctions. **Correlative conjunctions** also join equal parts in a sentence, but correlative conjunctions come in pairs. The common correlative conjunctions are *neither…nor, either…or, both…and, not only…but also,* and *whether…or.*

> Both her daughter and her son accompanied her to the clinic.
> *The correlative conjunctions **both…and** join the nouns **daughter** and **son**. Again, these words have equal roles in the sentence.*
>
> Neither the pathology report nor the CT scan indicated anything troublesome at this time.
>
> The medication affected not only his appetite but also his sleep.

CHALLENGE BOX

Test yourself on these sentences. Identify the conjunctions and see if you can determine the type of conjunction.

1. The patient complains of occasional dysphagia, no pain, odynophagia, ear pain, or any other problems.
2. Neither a gag reflex nor irritation was noted, yet he seemed tense and nervous.
3. He is suffering from significant disruption to his mood and difficulty with daily function.

I. PARTS OF SPEECH.

In the following sentences, identify each coordinating conjunction by checking the appropriate box under the words. If a word is NOT a conjunction, do not check the box under that word.

1. He was taken off Coumadin because he developed internal bleeding.

He	was	taken	off	Coumadin	because	he	developed	internal
☐	☐	☐	☐	☐	☐	☐	☐	☐

bleeding.
☐

2. He was anticoagulated with heparin, and a VQ scan was obtained.

He	was	anticoagulated	with	heparin	and	a	VQ	scan	was
☐	☐	☐	☐	☐	☐	☐	☐	☐	☐

obtained.
☐

3. Heart has regular rate and rhythm.

Heart	has	regular	rate	and	rhythm.
☐	☐	☐	☐	☐	☐

4. The breasts reveal no dominant mass, discrete calcification, or skin thickening.

The	breasts	reveal	no	dominant	mass	discrete	calcification	or	skin
☐	☐	☐	☐	☐	☐	☐	☐	☐	☐

thickening.
☐

5. Abdomen is soft and nontender without palpable mass or hepatosplenomegaly.

Abdomen	is	soft	and	nontender	without	palpable	mass	or
☐	☐	☐	☐	☐	☐	☐	☐	☐

hepatosplenomegaly.
☐

6. The patient was taken to the operating room, where anesthetic was given.

The	patient	was	taken	to	the	operating	room	where	anesthetic
☐	☐	☐	☐	☐	☐	☐	☐	☐	☐

was	given.
☐	☐

7. After the options were presented, the patient elected for a perineal urethrostomy.

After	the	options	were	presented	the	patient	elected	for	a
☐	☐	☐	☐	☐	☐	☐	☐	☐	☐

perineal	urethrostomy.
☐	☐

8. A midline incision was made and brought down to the periurethral tissue using blunt and sharp dissection.

A	midline	incision	was	made	and	brought	down	to	the
☐	☐	☐	☐	☐	☐	☐	☐	☐	☐

periurethral	tissue	using	blunt	and	sharp	dissection.
☐	☐	☐	☐	☐	☐	☐

9. The patient was prepped and draped in a sterile fashion.

The	patient	was	prepped	and	draped	in	a	sterile	fashion.
☐	☐	☐	☐	☐	☐	☐	☐	☐	☐

10. Although no fracture was clearly identified, a repeat study should be performed in seven to 10 days.

Although	no	fracture	was	clearly	identified	a	repeat	study	should
☐	☐	☐	☐	☐	☐	☐	☐	☐	☐

be	performed	in	seven	to	10	days.
☐	☐	☐	☐	☐	☐	☐

11. The patient was given a loading dose of Dilantin, but he did not respond to it.

The	patient	was	given	a	loading	dose	of	Dilantin	but	he	did
☐	☐	☐	☐	☐	☐	☐	☐	☐	☐	☐	☐

not	respond	to	it.
☐	☐	☐	☐

12. The patient was taken to the operating room, and he underwent a total knee replacement.

The	patient	was	taken	to	the	operating	room	and	he	underwent
☐	☐	☐	☐	☐	☐	☐	☐	☐	☐	☐

a	total	knee	replacement.
☐	☐	☐	☐

UNIT 3

Complete Sentences

COMPLETE SENTENCES – INTRODUCTION

The sentence is truly the building block of nearly all English writing. (Poetry would be one exception to this rule.) The very definition of a sentence explains why it is so crucial in communicating ideas. Let's begin by looking at what a complete sentence is.

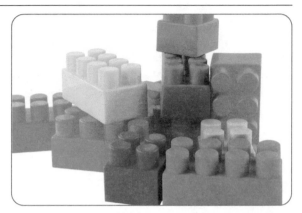

A **sentence:**

- has a subject
- has a predicate
- conveys a complete thought (it can stand by itself)

So, according to the definition, each sentence has a thing or person the sentence is about (the subject). It tells something about the subject (predicate). It contains a complete independent thought and can stand alone. So, each sentence is a neatly encapsulated, autonomous bit of information… Never thought of a sentence that way before? They are powerful tools and ones that you use well every day. Unfortunately, there are quite a few "pretenders" out there that look like sentences but don't meet all of the criteria.

SENTENCE FRAGMENTS

Keep the definition of a sentence in mind—a sentence must have a subject, a predicate, and must convey a complete thought. Problems can occur when any one of the three parts is missing or incomplete:

- If a sentence is missing a subject, it is not a complete sentence.
- If a sentence is missing a predicate, it is not a complete sentence.
- If a sentence does not convey a complete thought while standing alone, it is not a complete sentence.

To be proficient at identifying complete sentences, you should get in the habit of identifying and isolating the **simple subject** and the **simple predicate**. First, isolate the simple predicate, which consists of the main verb (and its helping verbs) in the sentence. Once you have that verb, you can ask yourself, "Who or what is doing that?" Who is running? What is ringing? The answer to that question will be the simple subject—**John** is running. The **phone** is ringing.

So, once you identify the parts of a sentence, you can see if any of these vital parts are missing. If so, the sentence is not really a sentence… it is considered a fragment. A **fragment** is a phrase or clause that is punctuated and capitalized like a sentence but does not have the required parts of a complete sentence.

FRAGMENTS CAN BE CAUSED BY A MISSING SUBJECT:

Came in for blood pressure check and cholesterol screening.
This fragment does not have a subject (the who or what it is about).

The patient came in for blood pressure check and cholesterol screening.
With the addition of a noun, it is now a complete sentence.

I. **MULTIPLE CHOICE.**
   For each of the following sentence fragments, mark the reason why the item is a fragment.

1. The results from the CBC and the ABG.
   - ○ missing subject
   - ○ missing predicate
   - ○ has subject and predicate, but is an incomplete thought

2. The patient, along with her accompanying relatives from out of town.
   - ○ missing subject
   - ○ missing predicate
   - ○ has subject and predicate, but is an incomplete thought

3. After he spent many hours applying a cold compress.
   - ○ missing subject
   - ○ missing predicate
   - ○ has subject and predicate, but is an incomplete thought

4. Replaced bandages often to avoid infection.
   - ○ missing subject
   - ○ missing predicate
   - ○ has subject and predicate, but is an incomplete thought

5. Because she injured the adductor magnus.
   - ○ missing subject
   - ○ missing predicate
   - ○ has subject and predicate, but is an incomplete thought

6. Prepped the patient in the usual manner.
   - ○ missing subject
   - ○ missing predicate
   - ○ has subject and predicate, but is an incomplete thought

7. Called to report the accident before entering the emergency room.
   - ○ missing subject
   - ○ missing predicate
   - ○ has subject and predicate, but is an incomplete thought

8. The patient with the severe case of hypotension.
   - ○ missing subject
   - ○ missing predicate
   - ○ has subject and predicate, but is an incomplete thought

9. Because we allowed the patient to contact his physician as needed.
   - ○ missing subject
   - ○ missing predicate
   - ○ has subject and predicate, but is an incomplete thought

10. Diagnosed her with bronchitis and warned her again about the risks of smoking.
    - ○ missing subject
    - ○ missing predicate
    - ○ has subject and predicate, but is an incomplete thought

FIXING FRAGMENTS

Once you have identified **why** a fragment is a fragment, making it into a complete sentence is usually pretty simple. If you add in the missing element(s), you can generally create a good, complete sentence without having to do much rearrangement.

A complete blood count with differentials.
This is missing a predicate. If you add a predicate the sentence becomes complete.

A complete blood count with differentials...
...revealed the problem.
...was ordered right away.
...arrived from the lab today.

There are many ways to make fragments into complete sentences. If you have a subject and predicate but the fragment does not express a complete thought that can stand alone, you can make a complete sentence by adding or removing words so that the dependent clause is no longer dependent upon anything.

When the patient arrived with an elevated heart rate.
*This has a subject (patient) and a predicate (arrived), but the word **when** makes this clause dependent. If this word is removed, the clause is now independent (which makes it a sentence).*

The patient arrived with an elevated heart rate.
Or you can add words to connect the dependent clause to an independent clause.
When the patient arrived with an elevated heart rate, the nurse recorded all of his vitals.
The physician ordered a complete physical exam when the patient arrived with an elevated heart rate.

I. MULTIPLE CHOICE.
Choose the item that is a complete sentence.

1.
- ⃝ The patient relaxed.
- ⃝ While relaxing on the reclined exam table.
- ⃝ The patient, now relaxed and under control.

2.
- ⃝ Because the prescription was called in late.
- ⃝ The prescription from the physician at the outpatient clinic in Durham.
- ⃝ The prescription from the physician was called in late.

3.
- ⃝ When the elderly man was escorted to the exam room.
- ⃝ Escorting the man from the waiting room to the exam room.
- ⃝ She escorted the elderly man.

4.
- ⃝ Presents for assessment of a pigmented lesion.
- ⃝ The patient, after being assessed for a pigmented lesion.
- ⃝ The patient is being assessed for a pigmented lesion.

5.
- ⃝ Otoscopy shows right ear to be abnormal.
- ⃝ Otoscopy of abnormal right ear.
- ⃝ Awaiting results of right ear assessment.

6.
- ⃝ Patient in no acute distress.
- ⃝ For a patient in no acute distress who is oriented x3.
- ⃝ Patient is in no acute distress and is oriented x3.

31

7. ⬭ Patient was advised 20 mg Lexapro increase.
⬭ Patient was advised to increase Lexapro to 20 mg.
⬭ Advising the patient to increase Lexapro to 20 mg.

8. ⬭ Anxiety and depression in remission.
⬭ Noted improvement with patient regarding anxiety and depression.
⬭ There is improvement in her mood.

9. ⬭ The patient is a 63-year-old white female with no previous cardiac history.
⬭ The patient's cardiac history, along with a detailed account of her family's cardiac history.
⬭ For a 63-year-old white female with no previous cardiac history.

10. ⬭ Hoping to be seen for GI assessment.
⬭ The patient was examined.
⬭ The patient's GI assessment, beginning with endoscopy.

RUN-ONS AND COMMA SPLICES

The term *run-on sentence* is a general term that comprises several common sentence structure mistakes. From the definition of a sentence that was presented a couple of pages ago, we can look at why run-on sentences are incorrect, what makes a sentence(s) a run-on, and how to correct run-on sentences.

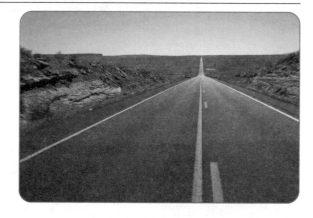

Remember, a sentence:

- has a subject
- has a predicate
- conveys a complete thought (it can stand by itself)

Most run-on sentences are simply due to a lack of proper punctuation. By definition a **run-on sentence** is two or more sentences (independent clauses) that are connected without any punctuation.

The patient says the symptoms are much improved he has no side effects of the medication.
You have two independent clauses that each could stand alone, but they are connected without any punctuation. This is a run-on sentence.

Run-ons like this can really only be corrected in one of two ways—you can join the two clauses or you can separate the two clauses.

> The patient says the symptoms are much improved. He has no side effects of the medication.
> *Since this run-on is simply two sentences, they could be separated into two sentences.*
>
> The patient says the symptoms are much improved, and he has no side effects of the medication.
> *The two independent clauses can be joined by a coordinating conjunction (and, but, for, or, nor, so, yet) and a comma.*
>
> The patient says the symptoms are much improved; he has no side effects of the medication.
> *If the two clauses are closely related in topic, they can be separated by a semicolon.*
>
> *There is a common thread in all of the corrections made: the run-on, which could not stand alone as a complete thought, can now stand alone as one sentence or two separate sentences.*

If you were going to splice two pieces of the electrical cord on your toaster together, you would not use clear cellophane tape. Cellophane tape is the wrong tool for the job. That splice would cause a health and fire hazard. Similarly, when you go to splice two independent clauses together, you do not use a comma. It, too, is the wrong tool for the job.

Often, comma splices are grouped in with run-on sentences because they basically have the same result—a structure that cannot stand alone. A **comma splice** is a sentence that is created by joining two independent clauses with a comma.

> The patient has a 150+ pack-year history of smoking, he notes a positive PPD in the past.
> *You have two independent clauses that could each stand alone, but they are connected with a comma. This is a comma splice.*
>
> The patient has a 150+ pack-year history of smoking, and he notes a positive PPD in the past.
> *Again, the two independent clauses can be joined by a coordinating conjunction and a comma.*
>
> The patient has a 150+ pack-year history of smoking. He notes a positive PPD in the past.
> *The two independent clauses can be separated by a period.*
>
> *Note: these sentences should not be joined by a semicolon because the smoking and the PPD are not closely related topics.*

The most common comma splice you will see is the use of a comma and a conjunctive adverb to join two independent clauses. Some common conjunctive adverbs are *however, also, likewise, therefore, similarly, nonetheless, indeed,* and *consequently.* These **cannot** join two independent clauses, even with the help of a comma! The clauses must be separated by a semicolon or a period.

> She was complaining of feeling hungry and had improving bowel sounds, however, there was still some left upper quadrant and epigastric tenderness.
> *This is incorrect. These independent clauses need to be separated correctly (period or semicolon) or joined correctly (comma and a coordinating conjunction).*
>
> She was complaining of feeling hungry and had improving bowel sounds; however, there was still some left upper quadrant and epigastric tenderness.
> OR

She was complaining of feeling hungry and had improving bowel sounds, but there was still some left upper quadrant and epigastric tenderness.

I. MULTIPLE CHOICE.
Choose the best answer.

1. The patient is a diabetic when he arrived he complained of extreme fatigue.
   ○ Run-on
   ○ Comma splice
   ○ Complete sentence

2. After checking his vitals, the physician ordered a sedative for the patient.
   ○ Run-on
   ○ Comma splice
   ○ Complete sentence

3. According to them, approximately 3 days prior to admission she fell in her bathroom, and she had fallen from bed about 10 days prior to that.
   ○ Run-on
   ○ Comma splice
   ○ Complete sentence

4. The patient has noted 2 purplish spots on his left foot, primarily his great and second toes, these spots are tender to palpation.
   ○ Run-on
   ○ Comma splice
   ○ Complete sentence

5. Having obtained informed consent, the patient was taken to the operating room and placed in a dorsal low lithotomy position, this was after he underwent general endotracheal anesthesia.
   ○ Run-on
   ○ Comma splice
   ○ Complete sentence

6. The patient went to school, and when he came home around 4 p.m., he was noted to be drowsy and not walking well.
   ○ Run-on
   ○ Comma splice
   ○ Complete sentence

7. Normally, this patient walks on his toes and does not talk a lot he has some evidence of developmental delay.
    - ◯ Run-on
    - ◯ Comma splice
    - ◯ Complete sentence

8. Physical exam revealed narrowing of his colostomy and I was unable to pass a finger below the fascia he therefore now presents for planned revision of his colostomy.
    - ◯ Run-on
    - ◯ Comma splice
    - ◯ Complete sentence

9. It was felt that in order to completely decompress this segment, a separate mucous fistula and colostomy site would be more favorable by dividing this loop.
    - ◯ Run-on
    - ◯ Comma splice
    - ◯ Complete sentence

10. After general anesthesia was administered to the patient, Lacri-Lube was instilled under the right upper eyelid, a Fox shield was placed over the right periorbital region.
    - ◯ Run-on
    - ◯ Comma splice
    - ◯ Complete sentence

UNIT 4
Punctuation

PUNCTUATION – INTRODUCTION

If there is one part of the English language that aggravates and torments most people, it would be punctuation. While most language skills seem very artistic, punctuation seems almost mathematical. What is the purpose of punctuation? Believe it or not, it is meant to make dealing with language easier… although that does not always seem to be the case. Punctuation was first formally and consistently used about 600 years ago (when printing began to replace hand copying). To this day, it is used to allow writers to convey their thoughts with precision. Punctuation can be used to remove confusion, signal pauses and stops, create inflection, and add meaning to writing. It allows the reader to absorb the language the way the writer intended. Without the proper punctuation, our language would be even more difficult than it already is.

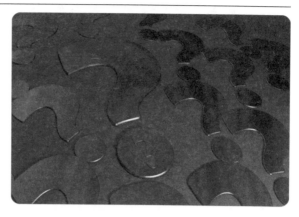

> **Jake picked up cream cheese and sugar from the store.**

According to the punctuation in this sentence, Jake bought two items: cream cheese and sugar. It sounds like Jake is planning on baking something. With the addition of commas, Jake's list changes.

> **Jake picked up cream, cheese, and sugar from the store.**

Jake now has three items that he got from the store: cream, cheese, and sugar. He may still be baking, but his ingredients are certainly different. The presence, absence, or position of punctuation can have significant effects on the meaning of our writing.

In this unit, we will focus on the most important and common pieces of punctuation and their uses.

COMMAS WITH INDEPENDENT CLAUSES AND SERIES

Commas are the most commonly used—thus, the most commonly incorrectly used—mark of punctuation. One thing to keep in mind with regard to a dictator's use of commas: they are sporadically and incorrectly dictated in medical reports, and even more frequently, entirely left out. Therefore, the first rule regarding commas and editing is *don't trust the dictator's use of them.* Be certain, however, that you understand and can use commas properly as it is **your** responsibility to make sure that the punctuation in the report is correct.

Study the following uses of commas, and be sure that you are comfortable with your understanding of them before continuing.

Commas to join independent clauses

The term *independent clause* is a fancy term that means *a sentence.* A comma and a coordinating conjunction (remember F-A-N-B-O-Y-S) can be used to join two independent clauses.

> The patient seems alert. She is scared and distraught.
> The patient seems alert, but she is scared and distraught.
>
> An incision was made over the anterolateral aspect of the shoulder. The underlying soft tissue was dissected down to the deltoid.

An incision was made over the anterolateral aspect of the shoulder, and the underlying soft tissue was dissected down to the deltoid.

Commas to separate items in a series

Use commas to separate 3 or more items in a series. Remember, the items may be single words, phrases, or clauses.

The patient is without complaints of nocturia, hematuria, or pyuria.

Extremities were without clubbing, cyanosis, or edema.

Over the next three weeks he apparently was fatigued, not able to do much at work, and had started feeling dizzy.

Abdomen is soft, nontender, and nondistended.

Do not, however, place a comma before the first item in a series, and generally do not place one after the last item in a series.

The external, internal, and transverse muscles were also incised.

The head, eyes, ears, nose, and throat exam was normal.

The procedure, risks and benefits, and possible side effects were explained to the patient.

The patient understood these risks, asked questions, and signed the consent form.

In all the examples above, a comma appears before the conjunction preceding the final element of the series. This is the classically correct style and has become widely accepted and even considered "the only correct way" by many. Your account instructions will tell you if this is not the case.

Do not use commas when multiple words in a series are separated by *and* or *or*.

The patient was without nausea or vomiting or diarrhea.

History included syncope and dizziness and loss of consciousness.

Pupils were equal and round and reactive to light.

It is quite uncommon to see series dictated this way in medical reports. However, such series are occasionally used, and you should be aware of how to punctuate them.

I. PROOFREADING.
The following sentences may or may not have all required punctuation. Add the necessary commas to make each sentence complete.

1. She experienced fever, anorexia, weakness, and right-sided chest pain.

2. Social history revealed that he lives with his aunt and uncle, does not smoke or chew tobacco, and reported drinking to intoxication once a month.

3. Abdomen showed extensive scarring, scaphoid appearance, no masses or organomegaly, no tenderness, and normal bowel sounds.

4. Strength, sensation, and gait were normal.

5. The patient was told to follow up next week, but he reported he would be out of town on business for a month.

6. She had a gastrotomy and biopsy and ligation of bleeders.

7. She is status post cholecystectomy, appendectomy, and bilateral hip prostheses.

8. Extremities had no edema and good strength.

9. Abdomen was soft, gassy, and nontender.

10. The patient was afebrile and active, yet she was apprehensive about being discharged at this time.

COMMAS WITH INTRODUCTIONS

Commas used after introductory elements

Commas are used to set off an introductory phrase or clause from the main independent clause.

> Although she was complaining of pain in her thigh, her lower back is painful to the touch.
> **Her lower back is painful to the touch** *is the main clause. The introduction precedes it and is set off by a comma.*

Usually participial, infinitive, and nonessential phrases that begin a sentence are set off by a comma.

> Thinking he had several alternate medications, he stopped taking the Allegra.
>
> To improve his breathing, he sleeps on an incline most nights.
>
> A fairly long and arduous test, the cardiac stress test allowed us to observe the heart in different states of exertion.

Prepositional phrases used as introductions to a main clause are generally not followed by a comma unless they are long (4 words or longer).

> In the West trained physicians perform most medicine.
> *But*
> From the excessive amount and extreme color of the drainage, I suspect a URI.

Sometimes single words alone can be used as introductions. If the words *however, also, no, yes,* or *well* are used as introductory elements, they require a comma after them.

> However, the blockage does not seem significant at this time.
>
> Well, we will have to schedule the test for the week of Feb. 14.

CHALLENGE BOX

Test yourself on these sentences. Where would you put commas in the following sentences or would you not put any at all?

1. After a long and very intense exercise session, she felt as if her heart were pounding too hard to be healthy.
2. Since she was unconscious and could not consent to the surgery, her mother's consent was obtained.
3. Preparing for her scheduled surgery, she took her medications regularly.

COMMAS WITH NONESSENTIAL ELEMENTS

Quite often we add extra information that is not necessary to the basic understanding of the sentence into our speech and writing. We refer to this extra information as a **nonessential element**. It is nonessential because the essence of the sentence is fine without this element being there.

> The patient, a pleasant enough woman, is being seen today for a yearly physical exam.
> *The phrase **a pleasant enough woman** simply adds extra (nonessential) information to the sentence. Without it, the sentence would still be complete and make perfect sense.*
>
> The patient is being seen, today, for a yearly physical exam.
> *Because the sentence would make sense without the phrase, we can deem it a nonessential element. If they appear in the middle of a sentence, nonessential elements are set aside by using a comma before and after the phrase, clause, or word that is nonessential.*
>
> Six weeks of therapy, both cardio and strength conditioning, will have her range of motion close to what it was prior to the accident.
>
> The patient's gait, a bit unstable and still slower than normal, shows little sign of improvement.
>
> We talked with the patient's husband, a patient also well known to us.
> *Nonessential elements may also appear at the end of a sentence.*

Essential phrases and clauses **do not** get separated from the main sentence with commas because they are essential to the understanding of the sentence.

The finger that has the torn sutures is to be cleansed and re-stitched.
To check and see whether or not this clause is essential or nonessential, take it out of the sentence.
The finger is to be cleansed and re-stitched.
While the sentence is still a sentence, it is missing some very essential information: which finger? That clause is essential to the reader's understanding of the sentence because it contains specific information about which finger will be part of the procedure.

The patient's eyeglasses with the bifocal lenses give him a headache when he reads.
Again, this is essential to the understanding of the sentence.

The man who hit her with the car was transported by helicopter to a nearby facility.
Again, this is essential to the understanding of the sentence.

I. **MULTIPLE CHOICE.**
   Choose the sentence with the correct punctuation.

1. ○ For now, we will simply observe the patient and make plans from there.
   ⊘ For now we will simply observe the patient and make plans from there.

2. ⊘ Because the swelling has subsided, we will re-wrap the bandage.
   ○ Because the swelling has subsided we will re-wrap the bandage.

3. ○ Because he has been out of the country the patient has not been seen for his left thigh pain.
   ⊘ Because he has been out of the country, the patient has not been seen for his left thigh pain.

4. ⊘ After satisfactory spinal anesthesia was obtained, the patient was prepped and draped in the usual sterile manner.
   ○ After satisfactory spinal anesthesia was obtained the patient was prepped and draped in the usual sterile manner.

5. ⊘ The wounds that were new were then covered with a compressive dressing.
   ○ The wounds, that were new, were then covered with a compressive dressing.

6. ○ The patient a 26-year-old white male sustained a right distal humerus fracture in a motorcycle accident 12 days ago.
   ⊘ The patient, a 26-year-old white male, sustained a right distal humerus fracture in a motorcycle accident 12 days ago.

7. ○ Traction was found to be stable not to mention pain free, after the elbow was brought through a range of motion.

⊘ Traction was found to be stable, not to mention pain free, after the elbow was brought through a range of motion.

8. ○ A well-developed, well-nourished white male in no acute distress the patient seems very amiable and polite.

⊘ A well-developed, well-nourished white male in no acute distress, the patient seems very amiable and polite.

9. ○ The patient had a duplex ultrasound, that revealed no clots.

⊘ The patient had a duplex ultrasound that revealed no clots.

10. ⊘ Between the meniscal tear and the peripheral rim, a debrider was used to roughen up the interval.

○ Between the meniscal tear and the peripheral rim a debrider was used to roughen up the interval.

COMMAS WITH COORDINATE ADJECTIVES AND PARENTHETICAL ELEMENTS

Commas With Coordinate Adjectives

Often, people will use two or more adjectives of equal importance in a row to describe something. These adjectives are called **coordinate adjectives**.

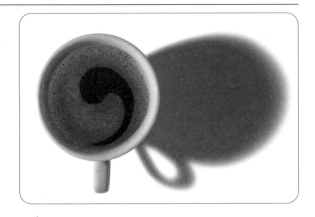

> The wound had a jagged, torn edge.
> *The adjectives **jagged** and **torn** are of equal importance. They should be separated by a comma.*

Not all adjectives positioned next to each other are coordinate adjectives (and, therefore, do not require a comma to separate them). Some adjectives have different degrees of importance in relation to the noun or pronoun they are modifying. To tell whether adjectives are coordinate, you can ask yourself two questions. If the answer to both of these is *yes*, then you have coordinate adjectives and must put a comma between them.

1. Could you put the word **and** between the two adjectives and still have the sentence make sense?
2. Could you change the order of the adjectives and still have the sentence make sense?

She is an independent, active female.

*Question #1- Could you put the word **and** between the two adjectives and still have the sentence make sense?*
Answer- Yes. She is an independent and active female.

Question #2- Could you change the order of the adjectives and still have the sentence make sense?
Answer- Yes. She is an active, independent female.

Since we answered yes to these, we see they are of equal importance and our comma belongs between them.

Presently he reports he is pain free and denies any tingling or numbness in the right lower extremity.

*Question #1- Could you put the word **and** between the two adjectives and still have the sentence make sense?*
Answer- No. Presently he reports he is pain free and denies any tingling or numbness in the right and lower extremity.

*Since we answered **no** to the first question, we don't need to go any further. These are not coordinate adjectives and don't require a comma.*

Commas With Parenthetical Elements

There are certain words we often use in sentences to add emphasis, order, or personal thoughts to the sentence. These are known as **parenthetical elements** (because they could be put in parentheses as well). When a parenthetical element is used in a sentence, it is set off with commas.

Her mother, to be honest with you, is not nearly as cooperative as the patient is.

This lesion, however, must be biopsied.

We contacted the patient's guardian, as mentioned earlier, to discuss the procedure.

TROUBLESOME COMMA RULES

Common Misuse of Commas With Dependent Clauses

One of the first rules of comma use you learn when you are in elementary school is the use of a comma and a coordinating conjunction (*for, and, nor, but, or, yet*) to join two independent clauses (sentences). This rule, however, often gets applied in situations where it should not be applied and creates a misuse of the comma.

Do not join an independent and a dependent clause or phrase with a comma and a conjunction the way you would two independent clauses.

Correct: She was able to perform a sit-to-stand activity with greater ease, and her standing balance reactions are improved.

> *There is an independent clause on each side of the comma so they can be joined with the comma and the conjunction **and**.*
>
> **Incorrect:** He came to us of his own volition, and appears to be in no acute distress.
> ***Appears to be in no acute distress** is a phrase and cannot be joined to an independent clause with a comma and conjunction. The conjunction by itself will suffice.*
> **Correct:** He came to us of his own volition and appears to be in no acute distress.

Common Misuse of Commas With Conjunctive Adverbs

Another common misuse of the comma is using the comma and certain transitional words (mainly conjunctive adverbs) to join two sentences. Some common conjunctive adverbs are: *also, however, likewise, nonetheless, therefore, similarly, consequently, so, otherwise.*

These words are not real conjunctions even though they are transition words. They can join two independent clauses; they just require different punctuation.

> **Correct:** The patient knew the risks of the procedure, and he opted to go ahead with it as soon as possible.
> *In this sentence, two independent clauses were joined by a comma plus the coordinating conjunction **and**.*
> **Incorrect:** The patient knew the risks of the procedure, however he opted to go ahead with it as soon as possible.
> *Conjunctive adverbs (unlike coordinating conjunctions) cannot be used with a comma to join two independent clauses. They require a semicolon (before) and a comma (after).*
> **Correct:** The patient knew the risks of the procedure; however, he opted to go ahead with it as soon as possible.
> *Or*
> **Correct:** The patient knew the risks of the procedure. However, he opted to go ahead with it as soon as possible.
> **Note:** *The conjunctive adverbs **so** and **therefore** do not require a comma to follow them when used in this way. This is one of the wonderful, mysterious rules of our language that makes it challenging to master.*
> **Correct:** The patient was looking forward to having the procedure; therefore he opted to go ahead with it as soon as possible.

I. **MULTIPLE CHOICE.**
   Choose the sentence that has the correct use of commas.

   1. ⬤ The patient was then prepped and draped in the usual sterile fashion.
       ◯ The patient was then prepped and draped in the usual, sterile fashion.

   2. ◯ The lining of the duct distally looked to have irritated frayed epithelium.
       ⬤ The lining of the duct distally looked to have irritated, frayed epithelium.

3. ○ Her left TM had a dry perforation, however, her right TM was okay.
   ◉ Her left TM had a dry perforation; however, her right TM was okay.

4. ◉ Skin showed crusting on the left pinna and scaly skin with early decubitus changes on the sacrum and ischial spines.
   ○ Skin showed crusting on the left pinna, and scaly skin with early decubitus changes on the sacrum and ischial spines.

5. ○ She had only a few teeth and some blotchy dark coating on her tongue from nicotine.
   ◉ She had only a few teeth and some blotchy, dark coating on her tongue from nicotine.

6. ◉ The patient is a quiet, well-developed young girl who is in no acute distress but is somewhat uncomfortable.
   ○ The patient is a quiet, well-developed young girl who is in no acute distress, but is somewhat uncomfortable.

7. ○ The patient shows decreased fullness, male pattern baldness, however, there are no visible scalp lesions.
   ◉ The patient shows decreased fullness, male pattern baldness. However, there are no visible scalp lesions.

8. ○ Exam shows a furious, robust, newborn infant.
   ◉ Exam shows a furious, robust newborn infant.

9. ◉ The hand and forearm were red and swollen with a cord up the right arm along the biceps.
   ○ The hand and forearm were red, and swollen with a cord up the right arm along the biceps.

10. ◉ Significant findings on physical exam revealed an ulcer on the ball of the left foot and very hypertrophic calluses on the balls of both feet bilaterally.
    ○ Significant findings on physical exam revealed an ulcer on the ball of the left foot, and very hypertrophic calluses on the balls of both feet bilaterally.

PERIODS

Periods are used at the end of a statement or complete sentence. When typing, periods (and all end marks, such as question marks and exclamation points) are usually followed by one space. In years past, two spaces was a common standard. In practical application, you will most likely be allowed to use either one or two spaces following end marks. However, be aware that you may be required to conform to the preferences of an individual client or medical transcription editing service.

Dictators will often dictate the periods in a medical report. Be aware of this and be sure not to type the word *period*. This is a very common mistake among new medical transcription editors because they are getting used to creating a document that is exactly what someone is saying. You also must be careful of this because dictators are sometimes wrong. They will either not put periods in where they need to be, stringing out several run-on sentences, or they will arbitrarily throw them in where they do not belong, creating incomplete sentences or sentence fragments.

The following is a reiteration of some common rules involving periods. This should be second nature to you.

Rule 1: **Primarily, periods are used to separate sentences.**

The improper use of a period to separate a sentence can create a sentence fragment. Likewise, failure to use a period where necessary leads to a run-on sentence.

Rule 2: **Periods are used in names and titles, such as Mr. and Mrs. or Dr.**

In this case, the period is always followed by only one space on your keyboard.

Rule 3: **Periods are used when typing medications in reports.**

This is a special circumstance unique to medicine, and you will learn this in depth in the pharmacology portion of your training.

I. **PROOFREADING.**
   Proofread the following sentences.

   1. Dr. Allen consulted on this patient. We informed Mrs. Smith that we would need to run several tests.

   2. There were no signs of injury. There seems to be no sign of a fall. We will have to x-ray to see the extent of the injuries.

   3. Some of his symptoms have subsided. I will prescribe him a new diet to address the others.

   4. They do not fluctuate with her weight. She has seen chiropractors, taken pain medications, tried physical therapy, and no conservative means have relieved or helped with her pain.

   5. His pulses are strong. His muscle strength is normal. Neurological exam: normal sensations.

COLONS

The colon is a piece of punctuation that has a more specific and focused purpose than many others. The colon is used to connect an independent clause to a list, explanation, rule, or quotation. The colon creates a harder "stop" than the comma or semicolon, and it does not have the variety of uses that some other punctuation has.

At this point, we will assume you know the basic uses of the colon. If you are not comfortable with the following uses of the colon, now is a great time to review them. There are many free grammar resources on the Web. The rules you need to be familiar with that we will not review are as follows:

- Insert a colon after a greeting in a business letter (Dear Mr. Chambers:)
- Insert a colon in expressions of time (3:32 A.M.)
- Insert a colon in specific account instructions after a subheading (You will study these in depth in a later module:)

Use a colon to connect an independent clause to a list.

> The patient has undergone the following procedures in the last three years: appendectomy, LASIK eye surgery, and cholecystectomy.
> *The independent clause contains the phrase **the following**, which is a signal that a colon and a list will come next. As a reader, you can generally anticipate what will follow a colon.*

Use a colon to connect an independent clause to an explanation or rule.

> At this point the patient's instructions are the following: do not work out with free weights for at least six weeks and ice the elbow liberally.
> ***It is generally acceptable not to capitalize a sentence that comes after the colon (like in this example).** If you have a situation where two or more sentences follow the colon, then you would capitalize each one. Of course, if a proper noun follows the colon, the proper noun will begin with a capital letter.*
>
> *The exception to this is when a rule follows the colon. If you have a rule that follows a colon, begin that rule with a capital letter.*
> There is one rule to fighting this disease: Always know what your caloric intake is.

Do **not** use a colon if the clause that introduces the list or rule is not an independent clause (if it could not stand alone).

> **Incorrect:** The patient is currently taking: Tylenol, prednisone, and Prilosec.
> *Because the introduction **The patient is currently taking** is not an independent clause (cannot stand alone), a colon should not be used here. In this case the list can be incorporated into one single sentence.*
> **Correct:** The patient is currently taking Tylenol, prednisone, and Prilosec.

I. **MULTIPLE CHOICE.**
   Choose the sentence with the correct punctuation.

1. ⊘ We dressed the site with Xeroform, sterile gauze, and an outer bandage.
   ○ We dressed the site with: Xeroform, sterile gauze, and an outer bandage.

2. ○ After the accident the patient reported the following, blurred vision, headache, and a sore neck.
   ⊘ After the accident the patient reported the following: blurred vision, headache, and a sore neck.

3.   ● I gave the patient my number one rule concerning prenatal care: You are no longer
        the most important person in your own life.

     ○ I gave the patient my number one rule concerning prenatal care, you are no longer
        the most important person in your own life.

4.   ● These are the medications the patient is currently taking: warfarin, Xanax, and
        Lopressor.

     ○ These are the medications the patient is currently taking, warfarin, Xanax, and
        Lopressor.

5.   ○ The patient told me he had a name for his most debilitating migraine, The Dark One.

     ● The patient told me he had a name for his most debilitating migraine: The Dark One.

6.   ○ She reported her most common reactions are: rash, itching, and wheezing.

     ● She reported her most common reactions are rash, itching, and wheezing.

7.   ● She said the single most important thing of all: getting better is up to me.

     ○ She said the single most important thing of all, getting better is up to me.

8.   ● She has had no recent travel, no ill contacts, no spoiled foods, no dysuria or
        increased urinary frequency.

     ○ She has had: no recent travel, no ill contacts, no spoiled foods, no dysuria or
        increased urinary frequency.

9.   ● I told her to call me if she felt ill.

     ○ I told her to call me: if she felt ill.

10. ○ We asked her to bring the following, her pain journal, her medications, and her unfilled
        prescriptions.

     ● We asked her to bring the following: her pain journal, her medications, and her unfilled
        prescriptions.

PARENTHESES

Parentheses are common in the English language, but they are pretty uncommon in medical reports. One reason they don't appear in medical reports very often is that parentheses are generally used as a nuance in writing; they indicate that the information within the parentheses is extra information and it is not vital to the sentence.

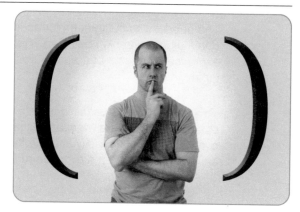

Medical reports usually contain important information with very little accompanying narrative. It is difficult to transcribe nuances, so parentheses are usually only used if the dictator specifies they should be inserted.

Parentheses set aside parenthetical ideas—those ideas that are not necessary to understanding the sentence. But as we learned earlier, commas can also set aside parenthetical ideas, and as you will learn later, dashes can set aside parenthetical ideas.

So how do you know when to use one and not the other? Well, as a medical transcription editor you will only use parentheses if the dictator indicates that they should be used. In general, however, parentheses denote an aside rather than an addition to existing information.

The patient's pain (so she told me upon arrival) is worst in the morning.

She has been taking an OTC pain reliever (it is Aleve, I think) for several weeks.
Parentheses do not require separate punctuation of their own, but standard punctuation and capitalization rules apply both inside and outside of the parentheses.

The parents wanted to speak to her as soon as she got to recovery. (The nurse explained to them that she would not be able to have visitors for several hours.)
In this case, the sentence inside the parentheses is a complete sentence of its own, so it is capitalized and punctuated like any other complete sentence.

When using parentheses, if you have a parenthetical idea *within* a parenthetical idea, you would use brackets inside of parentheses.

At the time of the incident, he was already in a cast (for a completely unrelated reason [I think he said he was seen in Phoenix for that injury]) and could not ambulate well.

I. PROOFREADING.
Proofread the following sentence.

1. The patient was being seen for an injured left ankle he suffered during a motorcycle accident (On a dirt race track, I believe.) This patient has a longstanding history of depression and has expressed thoughts of suicidal ideation [which seemed to peak about a year ago after his girlfriend died.] ,

2. This patient is a 33-year-old female who states that she began to have problems with her balance approximately 8 years ago (her complaints began after a head trauma.) Her complaints consist of fatiguing easily after prolonged activity and losing her balance during ambulation easily. (she has been a distance runner for years)

HYPHENS – LESSON 1

One strange little mark that causes a lot of trouble in the English language is the hyphen. A hyphen, unlike a dash, is not a punctuation mark. It is a spelling mark. This distinction can help us understand a little more about its use.

Hyphens with compound modifiers

The most common use of hyphens is to create compound modifiers. A compound modifier is created when two words act as a single modifier (adjective) for a noun. Unlike coordinate adjectives, which we learned create a series of modifiers, compound modifiers act as a single unit.

> The well-developed male is being seen for anxiety.
> *In this sentence* **well-developed** *acts as one modifier in its description of the word* **male**.
>
> She suffered a self-inflicted knife wound to the wrist.
>
> The 21-year-old female denies any history of alcohol abuse.

You will notice that in all of the previous examples, the compound modifier comes directly before the noun it modifies. Changing the placement of the compound modifier and/or the word it modifies can also change the rules of hyphenation.

Words and numerals are often combined to make compound modifiers.

> 12-ounce bottle
> three-piece suit
> 3-dollar fee
>
> *If the compound modifier contains a measurement, it is hyphenated* **only if an English unit of measurement is used**; *it is not hyphenated if a metric unit abbreviation is used.*
>
> 2-ton load
> 6-pound infant

4 mm incision
25 mg capsule
a one-third dose

Fractions are only hyphenated when they are used as adjectives. If they are used in other ways (like one third of a dose) they are not hyphenated.

If you switch the order of the noun and the modifiers, the role of the modifiers may change.

The 21-year-old female denies any history of alcohol abuse.
But
The patient is 21 years old and she denies any history of alcohol abuse.

*In this sentence, the modifier changed to a simple predicate adjective. It no longer acts as one unit describing the noun, so it is no longer hyphenated. Usually, if the **descriptors are not placed before the word they describe, they will not be hyphenated**.*

The patient is a full-time student.
But
The patient goes to school full time.
Again, the movement of the modifiers to after the noun causes the hyphen to be dropped.

Unfortunately, you must be very aware of the parts of your compound modifiers to ensure that you use hyphens correctly. If the word *very* or an adverb that ends in *–ly* is part of your compound modifier, you do not use a hyphen. The reason for this is the word *very* or the *–ly* adverb already signals to the reader that this is a compound modifier.

The patient claims to have a highly developed sense of smell.

She seems to have very limited movement of her left knee.

You do not use a hyphen if your compound modifier is preceded by an adverb.

The well-developed male is being seen for anxiety.
But
The very well developed male is being seen for anxiety.

This new-found mobility made her happy.
But
This seemingly new found mobility made her happy.

HYPHENS – LESSON 2

Hyphens are used when a prefix is added to a proper noun or a proper adjective. Likewise, words with the prefix *ex-*, *self-*, *all-*, or those with the suffix *–elect* are hyphenated.

ex-wife
pro-choice
anti-colonialist
president-elect
self-aggrandizing
neo-classical

Numbers are rarely spelled out in medical transcription editing, so you will seldom use the rule for hyphenating numbers. Numbers 21 through 99 are hyphenated when they are spelled out.

Thirty-six
Eighty-nine
Three hundred forty-five

Note: numbers 21 through 99 may be part of larger numbers, like 246.

Suspensive hyphenations are those that have two or more hyphenated words in which the second part of the modifier is used only once. These are essentially used to save space in writing, but dictators will often dictate them to save time.

The bandages were cut into 3-, 6-, and 9-inch links.
The hyphen is included in all of the modifiers, even when they are not complete.

She has a 5- and a 6-year-old child at home.

While this last rule is a combination and reiteration of earlier rules, it is being presented separately because of its prominence in medical transcription editing. There are several terms that get used in reports repeatedly and which, depending upon how they are used, may or may not be hyphenated.

The terms followup/follow-up/follow up are commonly dictated in the medical field. When it is being used as a compound modifier, it will be hyphenated. It has also become acceptable (and more popular in medical transcription editing) to write the compound modifier as one word. When it is used as a noun, the term is generally written as one word.

We scheduled a follow-up appointment for Tuesday.
OR
We scheduled a followup appointment for Tuesday.

Follow-up/followup is being used as a single modifier describing the appointment.

We scheduled a followup for the next day.

In this case followup is being used as a noun.

If the term is being used as a verb (it is something a person is to do), it is presented as two words.

The patient is to follow up with us in one week.

She will follow up with her dermatologist.

This same principle can be applied to many other terms you use in medical transcription editing.

Her arthritis will **flare up** if she does not continue her medication. *(verb)*

There was a **flareup** at the site of the infection. *(noun)*

The doctor will **work up** the cause of her abnormal heart rhythm. *(verb)*

During his **workup** for this tumor, he was found to have an abdominal aortic aneurysm. *(noun)*

She used the treadmill to **build up** her stamina. *(verb)*

A **buildup** of plaque resulted in the oral infection. *(noun)*

She was told not to **step off** the scaffold, but she did and she slipped. *(verb)*

The site of the **stepoff** was visible on the MRI. *(noun)*

I. **PROOFREADING.**
    Proofread the following sentences.

    ex-husband

    1. The patient, a 26-year-old female, arrived today with her exhusband and her son.

    x-ray

    2. On her followup, we discussed the xray, where we noted a fracture.

    3. She was given an anti inflammatory for her sprain, and we will follow up to monitor her insulin-dependent diabetes mellitus.

    2-shot   *one-half*

    4. A 2 shot T-tube cholangiogram was then performed using injections of 20 cc each of one half strength Angiovist.

    follow-up

    5. An injection was ordered for the follow up appointment.

    6. There is a yellow-green discoloration at the site of the ecchymosis that radiates 2 cm in all directions from the site.

    7. This 12-year-old male presents with fatigue related to anemia.

APOSTROPHES – LESSON 1

Most of us learned the rules concerning apostrophes when we were in elementary and middle school. And while the rules remain the same, applying them in medical transcription editing adds a new level of complexity to these rules. A medical transcription editor must be able to use the context of the dictation to identify plural and/or possessive words in a very quick and accurate way.

We will begin with the simple rules and work through some of the exceptions and more difficult rules.

To make a singular noun possessive, simply add an apostrophe + s.

The patient's sister

The specimen's

An incision's length

The cerebellum's measurement

The paramedic's report

Most words that are singular that also end in the letter *s* (or the *s* sound) still follow the original rule: just add an apostrophe + s. In all of these cases, an additional *s* sound is created by the addition to the word. You can hear the additional syllable when you say these words aloud with the extra *s* at the end.

The mass's circumference

Her boss's phone

Chris's parents

The dose's effects

Dr. Wise's diagnosis

There are a few words that end in an *s* sound that would sound awkward if an additional *s* sound were added. In this case, simply add an apostrophe. These are rare exceptions.

Ulysses' adventure

Dr. Moses' friendship

For some reason, there is some confusion surrounding making plural words possessive. There need not be any confusion. To make plural nouns possessive, you only have two choices:

1. If the possessive word ends in the letter *s*, simply add an apostrophe.
2. If the plural word does not end in the letter s, then you resort to the original possessive rule (add apostrophe + s).

The treatments' effects

The x-rays' results

The fingers' range of motion

The physicians' conclusions

The children's section

The geese's pen

The women's meeting

CHALLENGE BOX

Test yourself on these sentences. How would you punctuate the possessive words in the following sentences?

1. She held the nurses hand while we injected the antibiotic.
2. He reportedly fainted in the teachers lounge.

APOSTROPHES – LESSON 2

If you have a business or an organization or a hyphenated word, you make only the last word possessive. If you have two nouns or pronouns that own a thing together, you only make the second noun or pronoun possessive.

The brother-in-law's tests

Durham County Medical Center's history

The Agency for International Development's newest proposal

Jack and Carrie's dog (Jack and Carrie both own the dog)

Jack's and Carrie's dogs (Jack and Carrie each own a dog)

Units of time, measurement, or currency used as possessives follow the same rules that other possessive words follow.

A week's wait

Two hours' notice

A month's pay

A meter's width

A dollar's worth

Acronyms also follow the same rules that other possessive words follow.

> The NFL's top running back
>
> ABC's newest anchor
>
> The DOD's latest report
>
> The CPAs' ledgers (in this case, there is more than one CPA owning ledgers)
>
> The DMDs' preferences (again, in this case DMD is plural and possessive)

When using lower case letters, if you want to make them plural, you can use an apostrophe to keep the reader from being confused. If you use capital letters you do not need to use apostrophes. Double-digit numbers are made plural by simply adding an *s*; single-digit numbers are made plural by adding an apostrophe and an *s*.

> She often confused f's for e's when reading.
> *The apostrophe minimizes confusion.*
>
> In the 1970s, this test required a lot of preparation.
>
> We compared the CBCs and could tell there had been a remarkable change.
> *In these examples, there is no need to use an apostrophe.*
>
> The serial 7's revealed evidence of abnormalities.

Some pronouns are possessive by nature. These are called **possessive pronouns**. The possessive pronouns are *mine, yours, his, hers, ours, theirs, whose, my, your, its, their, her*. Since these show ownership in their regular form, you **do not** use apostrophes with them. Do not confuse these with all other pronouns that require apostrophes.

> That is her scar. — The scar is hers.
>
> That is his box. — The box is his.
>
> *But*
>
> That gown belongs to someone. — That is someone's gown.
>
> The room belongs to nobody. — It is nobody's room.

When a prepositional phrase that begins with the word *of* and contains a possessive noun or pronoun is dictated, the transcription editor may wish to revise it to remove awkwardness (unless account instructions prohibit editing of this type).

Original: His cast was removed by a friend of his sister's physician.
The phrasing is awkward and may complicate the transcription editing. This could be revised for clarity.
Revised: His cast was removed by the physician of a friend of his sister.

Original: He was in contact with one of her visitors' chaperone.
Revised: He was in contact with a chaperone of one of the visitors.

I. **MULTIPLE CHOICE.**
   Choose the best answer.

1. There were separate instructions for the (○ mens', ⊘ men's) examination.

2. No (○ ones, ⊘ one's) results will be returned before next week.

3. The nurse will return Dr. (⊘ Ross's, ○ Rosses) call after the surgery is complete.

4. After four (○ day's, ⊘ days') wait, the patient finally decided to seek help.

5. The (⊘ father-in-law's, ○ father's-in-law) diagnosis was well received by the family.

6. The (⊘ doctors', ○ doctors) conclusions were very similar to one another.

7. Dr. (⊘ Zenker's, ○ Zenkers') assistant brought his gown for him.

8. The instrument was used to measure both (○ kidney's, ⊘ kidneys') function.

9. The (⊘ GI's, ○ GIs) assessment was quick and conclusive.

10. Even if the (○ x-ray's, ⊘ x-rays) are clear, we will still order an MRI.

11. The (⊘ bone's, ○ bones's) surface appeared smooth and unaffected.

12. We received the (⊘ mother and father's, ○ mothers' and father's) consent for surgery.

13. The mother asked for her (○ childrens', ⊘ children's) medical records.

14. When the dog yanked on (○ it's, ⊘ its) collar, it pulled the boy down on his knee.

15. We gave the anesthesiologist an (⊘ hour's, ○ hours') notice prior to the surgery.

QUOTATION MARKS

In editing medical reports, quotation marks are not used very often (with the exception of psychiatric reports). When they are used, doctors will dictate them. In fact, they have to dictate them because as the medical transcription editor, you have no idea whether what the dictator is saying is a direct quote from somebody else unless he says it is. The most common instance in which quotation marks are used is when describing the patient's complaints. Because quotation marks are used infrequently and they are always dictated, they are relatively easy to use in medical reports.

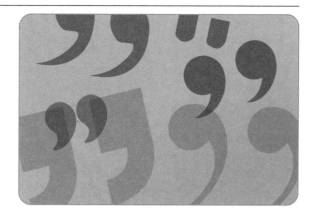

However, you must be careful when punctuating quotations because the punctuation for a quotation is often dictated incorrectly. You need to know the rules governing punctuation with quotation marks.

Rule 1: A direct quotation that is a complete sentence always begins with a capital letter. A direct quotation is followed or preceded by an introduction or identifier so the reader knows who is speaking. You will usually see introductions or identifiers like She said, He announced, I answered, Mary cried, John declared.

> Mary asked, "When are you leaving for the airport?"
>
> John said, "Give me all your kings."
>
> Harry answered, "Go fish."
>
> "We want some ice cream!" Sue and Nancy cried.

Rule 2: Periods and commas are always placed inside quotation marks. There are no exceptions.

> He said he had experienced "the jitters," but they were no longer present.
>
> "I feel like my legs are going to fall off."
>
> He describes the mucus as "mostly clear."
>
> The specimen, labeled "right fallopian tube segment," measured 1.5 cm in length.
>
> *NOTE–some of the direct quotations in the above examples are **not** complete sentences. That is why they are not capitalized.*

Rule 3: On the other hand, however, semicolons and colons are always placed outside the quotation marks.

> The following are described as "constant problems": swelling, pain on ambulation, popping, and clicking.

The patient complained of "feeling weak"; she was also describing dizziness.

Rule 4: Finally, question marks and exclamation points are placed inside the closing quotation marks if the quotation is an exclamation or question; otherwise, they are placed outside the closing quotation mark.

"Will I be okay?" she kept asking.

Will your specialist take a look at the "problem areas"?

I. **PROOFREADING.**
   The following sentences are completely without punctuation. Add all commas, periods, quotation marks, etc. as necessary.

   1. The patient described her issue as an unsteady feeling in my legs

   2. Stop Stop you're trying to kill me she kept screaming throughout the examination

   3. He described the color of the skin as sea green

   4. When asked about the headache, she said this is the worst pain I have ever felt

   5. The patient repeatedly asked how much will it hurt

UNIT 5

Capitalization

CAPITALIZATION – INTRODUCTION

Medical reports are pretty diverse documents when you look at them in their entirety. There is often an extensive narrative relating to history and complaints. There are often lists, quotations, steps (in procedures), and instructions. In order to maintain clarity and accuracy, a medical transcription editor must have a good mastery of the signals that readers use to aid in interpreting the written word. Punctuation, as we just saw, is one of our language's most important ways of signaling something to the reader—pause, slow down, stop, a list is coming, someone said this, this is possessive, etc.

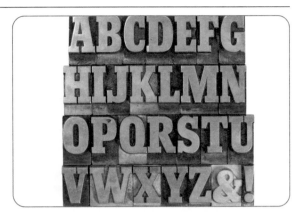

Capitalization is another way in which a writer (or dictator) can signal the reader. Only with capitalization, the signals are different—a sentence is beginning, this is a person's title, this word is important, this is an actual name of a specific group, etc.

Medical transcription editors have to know the rules of capitalization so they can apply them to the spoken word. It takes an understanding of the context of the dictation and of the conventions of capitalization to create accurate sentences and good reports. To make things easier, we have broken the rules down and will present a few on each page. You will be able to test your knowledge before moving on to the next set of rules.

CAPITALIZATION RULES 1–5

Rule 1: **Always begin a sentence with a capital letter. This acts as a signal to your reader that this is a new thought.**

> Some pain is felt on auscultation.
>
> The best course at this time is observation, and we will follow up in a week.

Rule 2: **Even though we just covered this rule, it is worth reiterating. When using a direct quote, capitalize the first letter of the quote if the quotation is a complete sentence itself. *If it is not a complete sentence, do not capitalize the first letter of the quotation.***

> When asked about her frequency, she said, "Every night I have to get up at least four times to go."
>
> She told me the pain is "like someone pinching me."

Rule 3: **Capitalize the first letter after a colon if there are two or more sentences *in the statement following the colon. If there is one sentence, phrase, or clause after the colon, it does not get capitalized.***

After examination, it seems the complaints are really twofold: To begin with, there is bilateral knee pain. Secondly, there is a weakness in her gastrocnemius.

I believe we have a single objective here: find the root of the pain.

Rule 4: **If the introductory portion of the sentence (prior to the colon) is very short and the heart of the material comes after the colon, then capitalize the sentence coming after the colon. If the introduction and colon are used to introduce a rule, capitalize the first letter after the colon.**

Always remember this: The point of the rehabilitation is to maintain function, motion, and strength.

I told her the first rule of recovery: Remove from your life that which initially caused the injury.

Rule 5: **If you have a list that is separated into outline form (lettering or numbering the items), the beginning of each item in the list is capitalized, whether they are complete sentences or not.**

PRIMARY DIAGNOSES

1. Severe right-sided heart failure.
2. Rheumatic heart disease.
3. Anemia.

CHALLENGE BOX

Test yourself. What letters in the following sentences should be capitalized?
1. she told me the feeling was "like a pinprick."
2. when considering options, take several things into account: do you want to spend a few weeks recovering now or a lifetime dealing with the pain? do you have a means of avoiding future damage to the site? do you have the support at home to help with recovery?
3. Of her elbow pain, she said, "the only good days I have are when I do not need to get out of bed."
4. CURRENT MEDICATIONS:
   1. aspirin
   2. warfarin

I. **PROOFREADING.**
   Proofread the following sentences. Insert capitalization as required.

   1. keep this in mind: the best medicines will only work if you are taking them religiously.

   2. Patient is Right Hand dominant. he has not had many blood draws in the left arm.

3. The patient was told to stick to the following diet: increased fiber, decreased dairy, and no sodas at all.

4. Some of the pain has subsided. she says it is now 3/10.

5. i have asked her to remain on the following medications: aspirin, beta blockers, and Lexapro.

CAPITALIZATION RULES 6–10

Rule 6: **Titles of people get capitalized if they are being used as part of or in place of a person's name. If the title is merely being used as a description, do not capitalize it.**

> The patient states she has worked for Congressman Aldridge for four years.
>
> He was brought here today by Pastor Allamance, his church pastor.
>
> He thought for a long time and said, "I think I can do this, Doctor."
>
> *But*
>
> I spoke with his pastor about possible counseling.
>
> We will ask his mother to come in.

Rule 7: **Capitalize a person's credentials when they follow the person's name, whether they are spelled out or abbreviated. Do not capitalize the credentials if they are just being used as a general reference rather than part of a person's title.**

> She was referred to us by Albert Pas, MD.
>
> We referred her to Steven Showalter, Doctor of Dental Surgery.
>
> *But*
>
> She was considering studying to be a doctor of dental surgery.

Rule 8: **The full names of companies, organizations, associations, government entities, foundations, and clubs are capitalized.**

> She claimed to have researched the illness through the National Institute of Health.
>
> When Sears closed down, she lost her job.
>
> The Department of Labor does not have good news for people in this patient's line of work.

Rule 9: *Department and clinic names are used very often in medical reports. This causes some confusion. We are going to break this rule into two parts to make it clear.*

Common department names that are being used as references to a general department are not capitalized. If the proper name of the department/clinic is used, the name is capitalized.

She was told that the wait at the emergency room was going to be several hours so she went back home.

She came to us from Central Coast Pain Clinic.

We released the patient on the grounds that he would follow up at the hearing clinic.

She was told that she would have to go to Cove City Hearing Specialties for her tests.

Rule 10: *There is a rule related to departments that is very unique to medical transcription editing. Doctors will often refer to a specialty as an entity in and of itself, encompassing the building, the people, and the department all in one. For instance, a doctor may say, "We will send the patient to Oncology." In this case, he is referring to the oncology department without saying so. When a department name is used in this fashion, it is capitalized. You should see a difference between this use (representing the department) and the common use of the specialty term.*

We referred her to Hematology and will follow up after her appointment.

*In this sentence, **Hematology** is used to represent the building, the people, and the department.*

When the patient arrived, she brought her hematology report from her visit last spring.

*In this sentence, **hematology** is just the specialty.*

We are awaiting results from Pathology.

The pathology results will be back on Tuesday.

CHALLENGE BOX

Test yourself. What letters in the following sentences should be capitalized?
1. Once we get the results from doctor Bailey, we may refer her to a pain clinic.
2. This patient suffered an injury to her femur during her work in the u.s. postal service.
3. This patient will be seen by cardiology immediately and I will consult with Jared Decker, md, facc.
4. If we get the pulmonary tests back, we will have her follow up with east wayne pulmonary center.

I. MULTIPLE CHOICE.
   Choose the sentence with the correct use of capitalization.

1. the consulting doctor ordered the patient to radiology for an immediate x-ray.
   ○ The consulting Doctor ordered the patient to Radiology for an immediate X-ray.
   ○ The consulting doctor ordered the patient to Radiology for an immediate x-ray.
   ○ The consulting doctor ordered the patient to radiology for an immediate x-ray.

2. at this time we will ask the patient to follow up with dr. alec at the podiatry clinic.
   ○ At this time, we will ask the patient to follow up with Dr. Alec at the Podiatry Clinic.
   ○ At this time, we will ask the patient to follow up with dr. Alec at the podiatry clinic.
   ○ At this time, we will ask the patient to follow up with Dr. Alec at the podiatry clinic.

3. he was ordered to follow a diet recommended by the american dietetic association.
   ○ He was ordered to follow a diet recommended by the American Dietetic Association.
   ○ he was ordered to follow a diet recommended by the American Dietetic Association.
   ○ He was ordered to follow a diet recommended by the American dietetic association.

4. the patient had been escorted to us from early dawn mental health by officer mason.
   ○ The patient had been escorted to us from Early Dawn mental health by officer Mason.
   ○ The patient had been escorted to us from early dawn mental health by Officer Mason.
   ○ The patient had been escorted to us from Early Dawn Mental Health by Officer Mason.

5. the patient presents today with an injury she received while working for the city.
   ○ The patient presents today with an injury she received while working for the city.
   ○ The patient presents today with an injury she received while working for the City.
   ○ The patient presents today with an injury she received while working for The City.

CAPITALIZATION RULES 11–14

Rule 11: **Days of the week, months of the year, holidays, and religious observances are capitalized. Seasons of the year are not capitalized.**

> We will see her back on the first Monday in June.
>
> She had a severe bout of depression when she was home for Christmas.
>
> She said she changed her diet drastically during Lent.
>
> The patient was seen in this clinic last spring.

Rule 12: **Directions on a compass do not get capitalized when they are referring to cardinal directions. However, if the direction is being used as a place (the South, the Midwest), then it should be capitalized.**

This patient arrived with his family for vacation and this is their first trip to the Northeast.

She said the dry air of the West helped her allergies tremendously.

The clinic is 20 miles northeast of here.

She was headed west on the interstate at the time of the accident.

Rule 13: **Most acronyms and initialisms are capitalized. However, there are some that have become common nouns through usage (scuba, radar). The words that the acronym comes from are not capitalized unless they are proper nouns.**

She was rushed to the CICU upon arrival.

but

She was rushed to the cardiac intensive care unit upon arrival.

The technique was recently approved by the ARA.

The technique was recently approved by the Academy of Rehabilitative Audiology.

In this case, the words that create the acronym also stand as a proper noun in their expanded form.

Rule 14: **Races (and sometimes nationalities) are frequently used in medical reports. Races, nationalities, religions, and tribes are capitalized. The exception to this rule is when the words** white **or** black **are used to describe a person's race (this is often the case in medical reports). If a person's race is designated white or black, the word is** not **capitalized.**

The patient is an elderly Caucasian man, an established patient.

She is an African American female, age 12, who presents with wheezing and cough.

Patient is a white male in no acute distress.

CHALLENGE BOX

Test yourself. What letters in the following sentences should be capitalized?
1. Tick-borne diseases like this are not uncommon in the north this time of year.
2. The patient has been exposed to severe acute respiratory syndrome, also known as sars.
3. She is a hispanic woman from a town east of columbia, south carolina.
4. If her progress continues, we will see her in july and then not again until fall.

I. TRUE/FALSE.
The capitalization in the following sentences is correct: true or false?

1. The child was transferred to the nicu on Monday, January 4.
   - ○ true
   - ○ false

2. She claimed they moved here from the Midwest last fall.
   - ○ true
   - ○ false

3. He is an alert, feisty hispanic male infant.
   - ○ true
   - ○ false

4. The patient, a white female in no acute distress, received the injury during a relay race on Easter morning.
   - ○ true
   - ○ false

5. Since last May, she has been treated for GERD (Gastroesophageal Reflux Disease).
   - ○ true
   - ○ false

UNIT 6
Agreement

AGREEMENT – INTRODUCTION

Have you ever wandered through a neighborhood and seen a house that just didn't fit in? You are not sure if it's the architecture or the building material—maybe it's the color or the landscaping. From the time we are young, we are trained to notice things that are different (remember the *Sesame Street* song, "One of These Things is Not Like the Others"?) We seem to work more comfortably and efficiently in patterns.

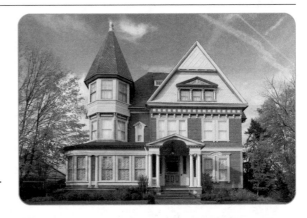

It makes sense, then, that our language is one of patterns. As we piece the words together to make sentences and the sentences together to make paragraphs, the patterns must remain the same. If something within a sentence breaks the pattern the writer set forth, it stands out to the reader like a brick Victorian in a neighborhood of pastel beach bungalows. When a sentence or paragraph has a structure in which all things follow the same pattern, it is said to be in agreement. The term *agreement* can refer to many things within a piece of writing:

- verb tense agreement
- subject/verb agreement
- pronoun agreement

In addition to these types of agreement, there are several elements of language that help ensure the patterns within a sentence or paragraph remain fluid and consistent:

- pronoun case
- pronoun reference
- modifier placement
- parallel structure

A piece of writing that is in agreement flows harmoniously and without hesitation. Agreement problems in spoken language, however, are not uncommon. As a medical transcription editor, you will be using the written and the spoken word at one time. As you edit medical documents, recognizing and eradicating agreement problems may be one of your jobs (depending, of course, on your account instructions).

TENSE AGREEMENT

When you were in middle school and high school and you were working through your English and composition classes, you were probably reminded to "Keep your verb tense consistent" by way of bright red marks in the margins of your essays. Whether you are writing essays or editing medical reports, you will usually utilize one main verb tense. This verb tense—past, present, or any other tense—is used as a reference for the time of other events in the writing. In other words, you may be writing in the present tense, but you can use the past tense in the same writing to signal to the reader that this event took place prior to the rest of the account. So maintaining consistent verb tense does not mean using the same verb tense all throughout your writing. It does mean that you must keep all references to a particular time in one tense, while using other appropriate tenses to signal changes in time within the text.

Her blood pressure **was** low, but it **is** now normal.
*The verb **was** is in the past tense, letting us know that at some point prior to the present (with the*

present representing the time of dictation), the patient's blood pressure had been low.
*The verb **is** is in the present tense and lets us know that at this point, the blood pressure is fine.*
Even though there are two different verb tenses in one sentence, there is consistency because the two do not conflict with one another.

Verb tense agreement problems occur when the writer uses different verb tenses when referring to the same time or when conflicting verb tenses create ambiguity.

When his cast was removed at the beginning of September, complaints consist of pain with weightbearing into the fourth metatarsal.
*There is certainly some problem with verb agreement in this sentence. The verb phrase **was removed** is in the past tense, but the second verb, **consist**, is in the present tense. This creates confusion about when the two events happened in relation to one another.*

When his cast was removed at the beginning of September, complaints consisted of pain with weightbearing into the fourth metatarsal.
By putting both verbs in the past tense, the reader now understands that both the removal and the complaints occurred in the past.

Sometimes the agreement problems, like the one in the example above, stand out and the reader's confusion is the first signal that there is a problem. Sometimes, however, the differences are subtle and a keen editing eye is needed to catch them.

The pain in the arm radiates to the elbow and moved down from the shoulder.
*The verb **radiates** (present tense) indicates that this is happening in the present. The verb **moved** is in the past tense. If the pain moved from the shoulder at some point in the past and ceased moving, then this could be correct. If the pain continues to move down from the shoulder as it radiates to the elbow, then **moved** should be changed to **moves**.*

How will you know which it is? Context, context, context. Your understanding of the report and the patient's condition will help you make the right determination.

I. TRUE/FALSE.
The verb tenses in the following sentences are in agreement: true or false?

1. Since the left anterior descending vessel is intramyocardial in its midportion, it was inaccessible for bypass.
   - ○ true
   - ⊘ false

2. Sterile dressings were applied and the patient was returned to the surgical intensive care unit in stable condition.
   - ⊘ true
   - ○ false

3. The patient had a significant smoking history but indicates that he will discontinue cigarettes 2 to 3 years ago.
   - ○ true
   - ⊘ false

4. The rectal exam is heme negative, and there was good sphincter tone and no masses.
   - ○ true
   - ⊘ false

5. The patient was discharged to home, and she will contact us if she needs assistance.
   - ⊘ true
   - ○ false

6. This patient is a 71-year-old Caucasian man who has smoked for 20 years.
   - ⊘ true
   - ○ false

7. The patient smokes a pipe and rarely had drunk alcohol.
   - ○ true
   - ⊘ false

8. The patient was unable to recognize her parents in the hallway and was using abusive language in attempts to be free of her restraints.
   - ⊘ true
   - ○ false

9. The patient continues to be followed in the SICU with a ventriculostomy and supportive care and her neurological status remained stable.
   ○ true
   ⊘ false

10. The patient was taken to the operating room, placed in a supine position, and anesthesia is being induced with infiltration of 1 lidocaine with 1:100,000 epinephrine, and IV sedation.
    ○ true
    ⊘ false

SUBJECT/VERB AGREEMENT

As children, we pick up on the subtleties of language through imitation and trial and error. You may hear a young child say, "You swims good." It is cute when a kid says it. It is not cute when an adult says it… or worse yet, writes or types it. Children will make mistakes when they try to create impromptu sentences because they are quickly (without thought) putting subjects and predicates together. They have not yet learned that certain subjects require certain verbs so the two will agree in number.

Since we will be using the terms *subject* and *predicate* over and over, let's review them:

Subject – What or whom the sentence is about. This person or thing will *do* or *be* something (contains a noun or pronoun).

Predicate – Word or words that tell what the subject is doing or being (contains the verb).

Creating simple sentences has become second nature to us and requires little thought on our part. We add a subject and a verb together and we automatically make the subject and the verb agree.

> The patient complains.
> *The singular subject **patient** agrees with the verb **complains**. We would be able to tell if they did not agree simply by the way they sound.*
>
> The patients complains.
> *This does not require understanding much about subject/verb agreement to understand that it is incorrect. But knowing **why** there is an agreement problem is required to correct some more complex sentences…sounding right is not always the best way.*

The problems that medical transcription editors confront regarding subject/verb agreement usually arise when sentences have compound subjects, phrases that intervene between the subject and the verb, or indefinite pronouns as the subject.

Anytime two or more nouns or pronouns make up the subject of a sentence and are connected by the word *and*, the subject becomes plural and will require a plural verb. If you remember back to your fifth grade math class, you will recall that the word *and* means to add. Similarly, in a sentence with *and* between the subjects, you are adding them together.

The patient and his 3-year-old brother take the same medications.

If multiple subjects are separated by *or* or *nor*, the subjects are being separated (rather than added together) and the verb will agree with the noun or pronoun that appears closest to the verb in the sentence.

Neither the laceration nor the fracture requires surgery.
*The nouns **laceration** and **fracture** are separated by the word nor. **Fracture** is the closest noun to the verb, so the verb must agree with **fracture**.*
A fracture requires.

Neither the laceration nor the fractures require surgery.
*If we make the word **fracture** plural, then the verb must change to accommodate the plural subject.*
Fractures require.

Understanding and identifying the subject and the verb in a sentence is required to ensure agreement between the two. If a phrase intervenes between the subject and the verb, make sure the verb agrees with the subject (and not with any part of the intervening phrase).

The patient, along with his parents, was taken to the recovery room.
***Patient**, not **parents**, is the subject of the sentence.*
The patient was taken.

Similarly, the subject of a sentence can **never** be in a prepositional phrase. (If you don't remember what a preposition or a prepositional phrase is, go back and review.) Prepositional phrases often follow the subject of a sentence, but don't get confused and try to make your verb agree with some part of the prepositional phrase. In fact, if you can mentally "cross out" the prepositional phrases, the subject of the sentence will be clear.

Fulguration of endometrial implants was performed.
***Fulguration**, not implants, is the subject. **Of the implants** is a prepositional phrase and cannot contain the subject.*
Fulguration was performed.

An examination of the fractures in the digits reveals displacement.
*The singular word **examination** is the subject. The subsequent two prepositional phrases (**of the fractures** and **in the digits**) lie between the subject and the verb and should be mentally "crossed out." The verb must agree with a singular subject.*
An examination reveals.

Test yourself on these sentences. Which verb would agree with the subject(s) in the following sentences?

1. The patient, in addition to both parents, (is/are) being moved into a new room.
2. Neither the treatment nor the medications (has/have) affected the patient negatively.
3. A piece of the fractured eyeglasses (was/were) embedded in the cornea.

SUBJECT/VERB AGREEMENT WITH PRONOUNS

Perhaps the most difficult subject/verb agreement arrangement is when an indefinite pronoun is the subject of a sentence. An **indefinite pronoun** is a pronoun that replaces a noun without giving specific details about the noun it is replacing… it's indefinite. This ambiguity makes it hard to ensure agreement between the pronoun and the verb. Some indefinite pronouns are always singular, some are always plural, and some can be either, depending upon the context of the sentence.

SINGULAR	PLURAL	DEPENDS
each	several	some
no one	few	any
every one	both	most
anyone	many	all
someone		none
everyone		either...or
anybody		neither...nor
somebody		
everybody		
either		
neither		

The list is hard to memorize. Just remember, indefinite pronouns ending in *-one* or *-body* are always singular. The plural indefinite pronouns (several, many, few, etc.) sound plural so they are easier to recognize.

One of the monofilament sutures in the fascial layer (was/were) removed using a Kocher clamp.
Which verb is correct?
What is the subject? It can't be **sutures** *or* **layer** *because they are each part of a prepositional phrase.*
One *is the subject. It is singular. It requires a singular verb.*
One was removed.
One of the monofilament sutures in the fascial layer was removed using a Kocher clamp.

Something in the chest x-rays (reveal/reveals) acute disease.
Which verb is correct?
What is the subject? It can't be **x-rays** *because it is part of a prepositional phrase.*
Something *is the subject. It is singular. It requires a singular verb.*
Something reveals.
Something in the chest x-rays reveals acute disease.

Those indefinite pronouns that can be either singular or plural seem to give people the most trouble. When using these pronouns, you must know what they are referring to and figure out if it is being used as a singular pronoun or a plural pronoun. The context of the sentence in which it is used will let you know if it is singular or plural.

Some of the sutures were loose.
*In this sentence, **some** refers to the **sutures**, which is plural. Therefore, the verb must be plural.*

Some of the laceration was healed.
*In this sentence, **some** refers to the **laceration**, which is singular. **Some** means part of the laceration. Therefore, the verb must be singular.*

None of the symptoms have returned.
*In this sentence, **none** refers to the symptoms, which is plural. Therefore, the verb must be plural.*

None of the pain seems acute.
*In this sentence, **none** refers to the pain, which is singular. Therefore, the verb must be singular.*

A couple of phrases that often need editing in medical reports are *the number of…* and *a number of….* When these phrases contain the subject of a sentence, there are specific rules governing their use:

- When used as the subject, the phrase *The number of…* is singular
- When used as the subject, the phrase *A number of…* is plural

The number of staples is appropriate for this size wound.

A number of staples were used to close the wound.

CHALLENGE BOX

Test yourself on these sentences. Which verb would agree with the subject(s) in the following sentences?
1. Each of the pins (is/are) being examined.
2. Some of the discomfort (has/have) been alleviated.
3. A number of minor abrasions (was/were) present upon examination.

REVIEW: SUBJECT/VERB AGREEMENT

I. MULTIPLE CHOICE.
Choose the best answer.

1. The patient, as mentioned in other reports, (⦸ is, ◯ are) in no acute pain.

2. The collection of cerumen (⦸ is, ◯ are) causing hearing impairment.

3. The patient's thoughts of suicidal ideation (◯ is, ⦸ are) very detailed.

4. None of the stools (⭕ seems, ⊗ seem) to be irregular at this time.

5. Sutures or a butterfly bandage (⭕ appear, ⊗ appears) suitable since the wound is superficial.

6. Angulation of joints (⊗ is, ⭕ are) unremarkable, but patient complains of recurring pain.

7. A number of contusions (⭕ was, ⊗ were) apparent upon examination.

8. Some of the fracture (⭕ appear, ⊗ appears) to be from a previous injury.

9. The medication, in addition to the physical therapy treatments, (⊗ is, ⭕ are) sufficient at this time.

10. Something in the patient's arm movements (⭕ are, ⊗ is) causing a popping and creaking noise.

11. None of the lidocaine injection (⊗ was, ⭕ were) given at this time.

12. The sinuses and the left ear (⊗ appear, ⭕ appears) clear.

13. All of the soft tissue swelling (⭕ disappear, ⊗ disappears) with application of ice.

14. Crepitation of the lungs (⊗ is, ⭕ are) audible upon examination.

15. Some of the degenerative changes of the lumbosacral spine (⊗ seem, ⭕ seems) accelerated.

PRONOUN AGREEMENT

Luckily, once you have a good grasp of subject/verb agreement, pronoun agreement is a piece of cake. Because pronouns, by definition, take the place of nouns, they often occur in the same sentence as the nouns they replace. The noun that a pronoun refers to is known as its **antecedent**. A pronoun must agree with its antecedent in number (and gender, if applicable).

> The patient must see his doctor in January.
> *The pronoun **his** refers to **patient**, which is singular and, in this case, masculine.*
>
> The patient's parents have a history of high cholesterol in their families.
> *The pronoun **their** refers to **parents**, which is plural.*

While subjects and verbs must agree in number, pronouns and their antecedents must agree in number *and* gender.

Remember the rule governing compound subjects in subject/verb agreement? The rule applies to pronoun agreement as well. *And* between two nouns or pronouns makes the subject plural and *or* between two nouns separates them.

The patient's wife and daughter brought their records in for comparison.
*The pronoun **their** refers to both **wife and daughter**, therefore it must be plural.*

The patient's father or grandfather had his myocardial infarction by the age 40.
*The pronoun **his** refers to either the **father** or the **grandfather** (not both) so the pronoun must be singular.*

As with subject/verb agreement, a phrase intervening between the antecedent and the pronoun does not change the number or gender of the antecedent.

The laceration, as well as the bruises on the arm, has healed and has lost its discoloration.
*The pronoun **its** refers to the subject of the sentence (**laceration**), so it must be singular.*

The phalanges of the left hand show no restriction in their movement.
*The pronoun **their** refers to **phalanges**, so it must be plural.*

Pronouns do not always have nouns as their antecedents. Sometimes a pronoun can refer to another pronoun. If the subject of a sentence is an indefinite pronoun, a pronoun somewhere else in the sentence may refer to it. Review the chart of indefinite pronouns from a couple of pages back if you need to.

Some of the audible rales were concerning in their intensity.
*The pronoun **their** refers to the subject of the sentence (**some**), which is plural in this sentence. The prepositional phrase **of the audible rales** cannot contain the subject.*

Some of the catheter had moved from its original position.
*The pronoun **its** refers to the subject of the sentence (**some**), which is singular in this sentence.*

I. **MULTIPLE CHOICE.**
   Choose the best answer.

   1. The fractures of his tibia had (◯ its, ✓ their) origin in an automobile accident.

   2. None of the skin surrounding the abrasions had fluid on (◯ them, ✓ it).

   3. The daughters of the patient said (✓ their, ◯ her) father has a history of smoking.

   4. The vein was unharmed so it was harvested from (◯ their, ✓ its) bed.

   5. The left anterior artery could not be located in (◯ their, ✓ its) midportion and appeared to occupy an intramyocardial course.

   6. The pain was primarily in the anteromedial thigh and calf and (◯ they, ✓ it) increased upon exertion.

7. The patient's inconsistent spotting or pain continued until the 20-week period when (◯ they, ⊘ it) subsided.

8. The region of surgery, indicated by radiation therapy markings, had tattoos on (◯ them, ⊘ it).

9. The dissection was carried down to the fascia, and (◯ they, ⊘ it) was opened using Bovie electrocautery.

10. The vertebrae were clearly distorted by the tumor, and (⊘ they, ◯ it) were misaligned above and below the tumor.

NOMINATIVE PRONOUNS

Pronouns can be used in many places in a sentence and can perform several functions. They can appear as the subject of a sentence; when used this way, they are in the nominative case. The **nominative pronouns** are *I, you, he, she, it, we, they, who.*

Without giving it any thought, you use these correctly nearly all the time.

> She was brought to the operating room.
> *She is the subject of the sentence. The pronoun is in the nominative case.*
>
> They will call someone who can bring her to the emergency room.
> *They is the subject of the sentence and **who** is the subject of the dependent clause **who can bring her to the emergency room**. These pronouns are in the nominative case.*

The nominative case gives us problems when we have two pronouns or a noun and a pronoun together. If you say the sentence to yourself without the extra noun or pronoun, you will recognize the proper nominative case of the pronoun in question.

> **Incorrect:** The anesthesiologist and her discussed the surgery options.
> *If you drop **the anesthesiologist**, look what you are left with:*
> Her discussed the surgery options.
> *That is obviously not the right pronoun case.*
>
> **Correct:** The anesthesiologist and she discussed the surgery options.

The nominative case is used in comparisons that use the words *than* or *as.* Most comparisons leave words out at the end of the sentence (and if you add those words in, you can easily identify the proper pronoun case).

> **Incorrect:** The patient's wife is older than him.
> *In reality this sentence has been shortened. The word **is** has been left off the end of the sentence. If you*

*add the word **is** to the end, you realize this is not the correct pronoun.*
Incorrect: The patient's wife is older than him is.
Correct: The patient's wife is older than he.

Incorrect: His wife has not been a smoker as long as him.
*Again, this comparison in its complete form would have the word **has** at the end of it.*
Incorrect: His wife has not been a smoker as long as him has.
Correct: His wife has not been a smoker as long as he.

OBJECTIVE PRONOUNS

Pronouns can also be used as the object (direct object or indirect object) of a verb or as the object of a preposition. Understandably, pronouns used in this way are said to be used in the **objective case**. The objective pronouns are *you, him, her, me, them, us, whom, it.*

The patient called me.
Me *is the direct object of the verb **called**.*

She wondered whom she should see about her dizziness.
Whom *is the direct object of the verb phrase **should see**.*

When she awoke, the nurse gave her all three medications.
Her *is the indirect object of the verb **gave**.*

I offered his wife and him a few moments to confer.
Him *and **wife** are both indirect objects of the verb **offered**. If you said this without the word **wife**, you would be able to tell that **him** is certainly the right pronoun choice.*

The patient would not reveal to whom the threats were intended.
Whom *is the object of the preposition **to**.*

Highlights

Is the word *whom* giving you trouble?

Remember that *whom*, like *him*, is in the objective case (and they look alike, too). If you are wondering whether to use *who* or *whom*, try a quick trick. Answer the question or restate the sentence. If you answer with *him*, then *whom* should be used. Otherwise, you would use *who*.

With (who/whom) did she have contact in the last 48 hours?
*She had contact with **him**. Therefore **whom** is the correct pronoun.*

The patient's mother knows (who/whom) is coming to visit.
Him *is coming to visit the patient. WRONG! Therefore **who** is the correct pronoun.*

CHALLENGE BOX

Test yourself on these sentences. Which pronouns should be used in the following sentences?

1. If we can meet with the patient and (her/she), we can discuss possible treatment options.
2. I discussed the option of surgery with the patient and her husband, and she was more enthusiastic than (he/him).
3. The patient wondered from (whom/who) she may have gotten the virus.

POSSESSIVE PRONOUNS

The final pronoun case is the **possessive case**. These are much simpler than the other cases and really require only your attention to the use (or lack of use) of the apostrophe.

As we mentioned in the Parts of Speech unit, personal pronouns and relative pronouns do not require apostrophes when used in the possessive case.

> Hers is one of the clearest examples of an MRI that I have seen.
> **Hers** *is a personal pronoun that is possessive.*
>
> The team gave its diagnosis.
> **Its** *is a personal pronoun that is possessive.*
>
> She could not remember whose medications she had borrowed.
> **Whose** *is a relative pronoun in the possessive case.*

Indefinite pronouns in the possessive case **do** require apostrophes.

> She said **someone's** shoes were left on the stairs and caused her to trip.
>
> Her mother told me that she would not listen to **anybody's** offers for help.

I. MULTIPLE CHOICE.
Choose the best answer.

1. The nurse asked his wife and (◯ he, ⊘ him, ◯ himself) to step into the examination room.

2. A person as young as (⊘ he, ◯ him, ◯ himself) should not have prostate problems.

3. The patient was asked if he was the one for (◯ who, ⊘ whom, ◯ whomever) the bullet was intended.

4. The boy said that (⊘ his, ◯ him, ◯ himself) parents were not aware of their activity.

5. No one is more aware of the seriousness of the issue than (◯ her, ⊘ she, ◯ herself).

6. The people from the doctor's office called (◯ she, ◯ herself, ⊘ her).

7. Between the father and (⊘ him, ◯ he, ◯ himself), there was already a complex history of heart disease.

8. The patient asked the nurse and (◯ I, ⊘ me, ◯ we) to help him onto the table.

9. The patient's daughter of nine is taller than (○ her, ⦸ she, ○ herself).

10. She did not know from (⦸ whom, ○ who, ○ whomever) the original phone call came.

II. FILL IN THE BLANK.

Using the word(s) in the box, enter the appropriate term in the space provided. Terms may be used more than once.

1. When he arrived, he was as talkative as ___she___ .

2. In an effort to minimize movement, the patient and ___she___ were lifted carefully onto a stretcher.

3. A fight between her boyfriend and ___her___ caused her initial injury.

4. The patient called for help from work, where ___her___ heavy lifting caused a debilitating pain in her lower back.

5. Although the medication was ___hers___ , she claimed to have never actually taken any.

her
she
hers
herself

MODIFIER PLACEMENT

Since the integrity and accuracy of the patient's medical record is at the heart of the medical transcription editor's job, the MTE must be exacting. Perhaps nowhere is there more room for interpretive error on the part of the reader than when working with the placement (and misplacement) of modifiers.

A **modifier** is an adjective, adverb, phrase, or clause that acts as an adjective or an adverb… a modifier modifies something in the sentence. The importance of the **placement** of the modifier can be seen by looking at a couple of examples:

Taking several medications that affected her coordination, the doctor observed the patient carefully.

*The modifier is **Taking several medications that affected her coordination**. The question must be asked, "WHO was taking several medications that affected her coordination?"*

*In this case, we hope it was the patient who was taking the medications and not the doctor. Notice the modifying phrase is right next to **the doctor**. According to the placement of the modifier, it seems that the doctor is the one who was taking the medication.*

Inserting the IV and beginning the drip, the patient began to relax.

Again, there is some confusion in this sentence. Did the patient insert the IV and begin the drip? I hope not… that does not seem like sound medical practice.

How do we ensure that the modifier is saying exactly what we want it to say? Usually the **placement** of the modifier in the sentence can create clarity. When a sentence begins with a modifier, the thing (noun/pronoun) that immediately follows it should be the thing that is supposed to be modified. In our example sentences, this placement problem causes the confusion:

Taking several medications that affected her coordination, the doctor observed the patient carefully.

*In this sentence, the modifier is modifying **the doctor** because it is the thing that immediately follows the modifying phrase.*

This confusion can be alleviated by changing the sentence and the placement of the modifier.

The doctor carefully observed the patient, who was taking several medications that affected her coordination.

This is much better. There is no doubt who was doing the observing and who was taking the medication.

MODIFIER CLARITY

In an effort to simplify the modifier rules, we will list the most important ones here and give examples of each.

Modifiers at the beginning of a sentence

Make sure a modifier at the beginning of a sentence refers to the thing that comes right after it in the sentence.

Incorrect: Though legally blind, the construction site is not a hazardous place for the patient.

Correct: Though he is legally blind, the patient does not find the construction site hazardous.

OR

Correct: Though the patient is legally blind, the construction site does not pose a hazard for him.

Modifier proximity to modified words

Place modifiers logically next to the word(s) they modify.

Incorrect: The patient is a 58-year-old female with a sprained ankle weighing 125 pounds.

Correct: The patient is a 58-year-old female weighing 125 pounds, and she has a sprained ankle.

Limiting modifiers

Limiting modifiers should always go directly in front of the word(s) they modify. Limiting modifiers are *only, not, nearly, hardly, almost, just, merely, simply, even.*

Incorrect: The patient nearly had 3000 ml saline.
*In this sentence, the placement of the word **nearly** implies that the patient narrowly escaped having the saline.*

Correct: The patient had nearly 3000 ml saline.
*In this sentence, the placement of the word **nearly** explains that almost the entire 3000 ml of saline was given to the patient.*

Split infinitives

Infinitives are created by placing the word *to* in front of a main verb (to palpate, to puncture, to assess). Do not split up infinitives with long, intrusive modifiers. It will create an awkward sentence.

Incorrect: The surgeon planned to, with the help of an assisting surgeon, prep the patient immediately.
*The infinitive **to prep** is split by a long intervening phrase and the sentence becomes quite awkward.*

Correct: The surgeon, with the help of an assisting surgeon, planned to prep the patient immediately.

I. **MULTIPLE CHOICE.**
   In the following exercises, there are two sentences. Select the one that has the correct use of modifiers.

   1. ○ The sutures in the wounds that have been there for a week are ready to be removed.
      ⦸ In the wounds, the sutures have been there for a week and are ready to be removed.

   2. ⦸ Expecting the worst, the patient was surprised to see his blood pressure was 138/78.
      ○ Expecting the worst, the patient's blood pressure was a surprisingly low 138/78.

   3. ○ The patient was taken to the room with a wheelchair.
      ⦸ The patient was taken in a wheelchair to the examining room.

   4. ⦸ Describing the pain as burning and intermittent, the patient explained that the pain extends through the volar forearm.
      ○ Describing the pain as burning and intermittent, the pain extends through the volar forearm, according to the patient.

   5. ⦸ After thorough counseling as to the indications, procedure, and complications of the procedure, the patient was taken to the operating room on February 4, 2006, and a splenectomy was performed.
      ○ After thorough counseling as to the indications, procedure, and complications of the procedure, a splenectomy was performed on February 4, 2006.

6. ○ After the surgery, the patient was barely able to walk with any help.
    ⊘ After the surgery, the patient was able to walk with barely any help.

7. ○ The patient arrived with extreme pain in her workplace.
    ⊘ The patient arrived at her workplace in extreme pain.

8. ⊘ Soft and nontender, the abdomen seemed no cause for concern.
    ○ Soft and nontender, I had no concern regarding the patient's abdomen.

9. ⊘ This 50-year-old female patient with carcinoma of the left breast complains today of reflux.
    ○ This 50-year-old female patient complains today of reflux with carcinoma of the left breast.

10. ○ As a young child, I had seen this patient for acute appendicitis.
    ⊘ I had seen this patient as a young child for acute appendicitis.

PARALLEL STRUCTURE

It has often been said that good writing is a mix of art and science. While you, as a medical transcription editor, do not need the artistic abilities to write a great piece of prose, you do have to make sure that what you record is precise (in many ways—precisely what the dictator says and sometimes precisely what he meant to say, depending upon your account instructions). So your writing, while not original content, must be good writing. Much of a person's healthcare record depends upon it.

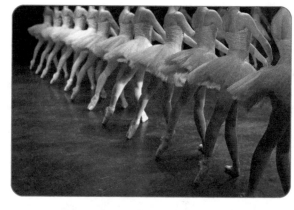

One of those rules that seems more science than art that governs the English language is that of parallel structure. Parallel means the same thing in writing that it does in geometry: having the same course, direction, nature, or tendency. You can look at two lines and tell if they are parallel or not almost immediately. With writing, of course, it takes a little closer inspection. Parallelism means that you have consistency in the patterns and structures in your writing—usually this means using similar forms of words, phrases, or clauses.

Incorrect: The bleeding was controlled, the hemisternum was elevated, and we exposed the internal mammary region.
We have three clauses in this sentence that need to be parallel. To make them parallel, they must be written in the same form. When you separate them, you can see that they are not in the same form:
The bleeding was controlled
the hemisternum was elevated
and we exposed the internal mammary region.

The structure that was set up by the first two clauses—the + noun + verb phrase—is broken by the last clause. It can easily be corrected by putting it into the same pattern.
Correct: The bleeding was controlled, the hemisternum was elevated, and the internal mammary region was exposed.

To maintain parallelism in a sentence, do not mix forms: if you use the infinitive form (*to* + verb), use it throughout. If you use the gerund form (*ing* ending on a verb), use it throughout.

Incorrect: The patient was advised to cut sodium intake, to increase exercise, and please chart BP daily for one month.
Correct: The patient was advised to cut sodium intake, to increase exercise, and to chart BP daily for one month.

Incorrect: Patient reports drinking socially, smoking daily, and occasional drug use.
Correct: Patient reports drinking socially, smoking daily, and using drugs occasionally.

When clauses are used in a sentence, their use must continue throughout (if in a series).

Incorrect: The nurse told the patient that she should get some rest, that she should drink plenty of fluids, and to use ice as needed.
Correct: The nurse told the patient that she should get some rest, that she should drink plenty of fluids, and that she should use ice as needed.

Medical reports often contain lists. If the lists are part of a sentence (as opposed to a vertical numbered list), parallelism should be maintained unless your account instructions say otherwise.

Incorrect: She reports pain during the following: lifting, driving, bending, and during urination.
Correct: She reports pain during the following: lifting, driving, bending, and urinating.

I. **TRUE/FALSE.**
   Mark the following true if the sentence has parallel structure or false if there is a parallel structure error(s).

   1. The patient reported that he tripped over the step, grabbed the railing, and fell down three stairs.
      - ⊘ true
      - ○ false

   2. The patient was congenial, alert, and the kind of person who does mind questions.
      - ○ true
      - ⊘ false

3. She reported the following symptoms: dizziness, headache, needing to urinate.
   ○ true
   ⊘ false

4. An epidural anesthetic, arterial line, and general endotracheal anesthesia were performed by the anesthesia service.
   ⊕ true
   ○ false

5. The lateral vascular pedicles were dissected down to the level of the endopelvic fascia, the peritoneum was incised posteriorly at the reflection between the bladder and the rectum, and I dissected the posterior vascular pedicles of the bladder.
   ○ true
   ⊘ false

6. The patient was started on IV antibiotics, the Foley catheter was inserted, and given IV hydration.
   ○ true
   ⊘ false

7. He is awake and alert, is voiding well now at a current level of 2 mg p.o. q.h.s., and is ready for discharge to home.
   ⊕ true
   ○ false

8. A horizontal linear incision was made in the right anterior neck, self-retaining retractors were placed, and dissection was carried down to the platysma.
   ⊘ true
   ○ false

9. The patient states that about a year and a half ago the pain began radiating into the left lower back, into the buttocks, into the posterior thigh, and the entire foot.
   ○ true
   ⊘ false

10. Thus, the patient was taken to the operating room where he underwent a left L5-S1 hemilaminectomy, diskectomy, and the foramen was enlarged.
    ○ true
    ⊘ false

ANSWER KEY

Parts of Speech

NOUNS AND PRONOUNS

CHALLENGE BOX.

1. **She** and **you** are personal pronouns and **what** is an interrogative pronoun.
2. **Everyone** is an indefinite pronoun and **her** is a possessive pronoun.
3. **These** is a demonstrative pronoun.
4. **That** is a relative pronoun that links the dependent clause **that landed here** to the word **plane**. **Its** is a possessive pronoun.
5. **Nobody** is an indefinite pronoun. **We** is a personal pronoun. **That** is a relative pronoun.

ADJECTIVES

I. MULTIPLE CHOICE.

1. pronoun
2. adjective - pain
3. adjective - region OR adjective - trochanteric region
4. adjective - region
5. noun
6. noun
7. noun
8. noun
9. pronoun
10. adjective - pain
11. noun
12. adjective - gutters
13. adjective - gutters
14. noun
15. adjective - compartment
16. noun
17. adjective - plateau
18. noun
19. noun
20. adjective - room
21. noun
22. noun
23. adjective - cautery
24. noun

VERBS

CHALLENGE BOX.

1. **Will call** is a compound verb and it shows action.
2. **Received** is an action verb.
3. **Does have** is a compound verb showing action. **Will send** is a compound verb and it shows action.
4. **Appeared** is a linking verb that shows his state of being (oriented). **Spoke** is an action verb.
5. **Looks** is a linking verb expressing state of being (good). **Will follow up** is a compound verb showing action. **Change** is an action verb.

ADVERBS IN ACTION

I. MULTIPLE CHOICE.

1. immediately
2. normally
3. somewhat
4. unusually
5. yearly

II. FILL IN THE BLANK.

1. return
2. return
3. had suffered
4. progressed
5. were irrigated
6. exaggerated

REVIEW: PARTS OF SPEECH

I. MULTIPLE CHOICE.

1. noun
2. verb
3. adjective - history
4. noun
5. noun
6. adjective - cough OR adjective - problems
7. verb
8. adjective - episodes
9. verb
10. noun
11. verb
12. noun
13. adjective - rash
14. noun
15. adverb
16. verb
17. noun
18. verb
19. adverb
20. verb
21. noun
22. verb
23. pronoun
24. pronoun
25. adverb

PREPOSITIONS

CHALLENGE BOX.

1. of the left lung
2. on admission
3. For that reason, by the hospital social worker
4. for a workup, of his suspected atherosclerotic peripheral vascular disease
5. to the descending portion, of the colon, on its antimesentery border, by electrocautery, along the white line, of Toldt

I. TRUE/FALSE.

1. false
2. true
3. false
4. true
5. true
6. false
7. true
8. true
9. false
10. true

CONJUNCTIONS

CHALLENGE BOX.

1. **Or** is a coordinating conjunction.
2. **Neither...nor** is a correlative conjunction. **Yet** is a coordinating. **And** is a coordinating conjunction.
3. **And** is a coordinating conjunction.

I. PARTS OF SPEECH.

1. none
2. and
3. and
4. or
5. and, or
6. none

7. none
8. and, and
9. and
10. none
11. but
12. and

Complete Sentences

SENTENCE FRAGMENTS

I. MULTIPLE CHOICE.
1. missing predicate
2. missing predicate
3. has subject and predicate, but is an incomplete thought
4. missing subject
5. has subject and predicate, but is an incomplete thought
6. missing subject
7. missing subject
8. missing predicate
9. has subject and predicate, but is an incomplete thought
10. missing subject

FIXING FRAGMENTS

I. MULTIPLE CHOICE.
1. The patient relaxed.
2. The prescription from the physician was called in late.
3. She escorted the elderly man.
4. The patient is being assessed for a pigmented lesion.
5. Otoscopy shows right ear to be abnormal.
6. Patient is in no acute distress and is oriented x3.
7. Patient was advised to increase Lexapro to 20 mg.
8. There is improvement in her mood.
9. The patient is a 63-year-old white female with no previous cardiac history.
10. The patient was examined.

RUN-ONS AND COMMA SPLICES

I. MULTIPLE CHOICE.
1. Run-on
2. Complete sentence
3. Complete sentence
4. Comma splice
5. Comma splice
6. Complete sentence
7. Run-on
8. Run-on
9. Complete sentence
10. Comma splice

Punctuation

COMMAS WITH INDEPENDENT CLAUSES AND SERIES

I. PROOFREADING.

1. She experienced fever , anorexia , weakness , and right-sided chest pain.
2. Social history revealed that he lives with his aunt and uncle , does not smoke or chew tobacco , and reported drinking to intoxication once a month.
3. Abdomen showed extensive scarring , scaphoid appearance , no masses or organomegaly , no tenderness , and normal bowel sounds.
4. Strength, sensation, and gait were normal.
5. The patient was told to follow up next week , but he reported he would be out of town on business for a month.
6. She had a gastrotomy and biopsy and ligation of bleeders.
7. She is status post cholecystectomy, appendectomy, and bilateral hip prostheses.
8. Extremities had no edema and good strength.
9. Abdomen was soft , gassy , and nontender.
10. The patient was afebrile and active , yet she was apprehensive about being discharged at this time.

COMMAS WITH INTRODUCTIONS

CHALLENGE BOX.

1. After a long and very intense exercise session, she felt as if her heart were pounding too hard to be healthy.
   After a long and very intense exercise session is a long prepositional phrase so it would have a comma after it.
2. Since she was unconscious and could not consent to the surgery, her mother's consent was obtained.
   Since she was unconscious and could not consent to the surgery is an introductory clause.
3. Preparing for her scheduled surgery, she took her medications regularly.
   Preparing for her scheduled surgery is an introductory phrase.

COMMAS WITH NONESSENTIAL ELEMENTS

I. MULTIPLE CHOICE.

1. For now we will simply observe the patient and make plans from there.
2. Because the swelling has subsided, we will re-wrap the bandage.
3. Because he has been out of the country, the patient has not been seen for his left thigh pain.
4. After satisfactory spinal anesthesia was obtained, the patient was prepped and draped in the usual sterile manner.
5. The wounds that were new were then covered with a compressive dressing.
6. The patient, a 26-year-old white male, sustained a right distal humerus fracture in a motorcycle accident 12 days ago.
7. Traction was found to be stable, not to mention pain free, after the elbow was brought through a range of motion.
8. A well-developed, well-nourished white male in no acute distress, the patient seems very amiable and polite.
9. The patient had a duplex ultrasound that revealed no clots.
10. Between the meniscal tear and the peripheral rim, a debrider was used to roughen up the interval.

TROUBLESOME COMMA RULES

I. MULTIPLE CHOICE.

1. The patient was then prepped and draped in the usual sterile fashion.

2. The lining of the duct distally looked to have irritated, frayed epithelium.

3. Her left TM had a dry perforation; however, her right TM was okay.

4. Skin showed crusting on the left pinna and scaly skin with early decubitus changes on the sacrum and ischial spines.

5. She had only a few teeth and some blotchy, dark coating on her tongue from nicotine.

6. The patient is a quiet, well-developed young girl who is in no acute distress but is somewhat uncomfortable.

7. The patient shows decreased fullness, male pattern baldness. However, there are no visible scalp lesions.

8. Exam shows a furious, robust newborn infant.

9. The hand and forearm were red and swollen with a cord up the right arm along the biceps.

10. Significant findings on physical exam revealed an ulcer on the ball of the left foot and very hypertrophic calluses on the balls of both feet bilaterally.

PERIODS

I. PROOFREADING.

1. Dr . Allen consulted on this patient . We informed Mrs . Smith that we would need to run several tests .

2. There were no signs of injury . There seems to be no sign of a fall . We will have to x-ray to see the extent of the injuries .

3. Some of his symptoms have subsided . I will prescribe him a new diet to address the others .

4. They do not fluctuate with her weight. She has seen chiropractors, taken pain medications, tried physical therapy, and no conservative means have relieved or helped with her pain ; .

5. His pulses are strong . His muscle strength is normal . Neurological exam: normal sensations.

COLONS

I. MULTIPLE CHOICE.

1. We dressed the site with Xeroform, sterile gauze, and an outer bandage.

2. After the accident the patient reported the following: blurred vision, headache, and a sore neck.

3. I gave the patient my number one rule concerning prenatal care: You are no longer the most important person in your own life.

4. These are the medications the patient is currently taking: warfarin, Xanax, and Lopressor.

5. The patient told me he had a name for his most debilitating migraine: The Dark One.

6. She reported her most common reactions are rash, itching, and wheezing.

7. She said the single most important thing of all: getting better is up to me.

8. She has had no recent travel, no ill contacts, no spoiled foods, no dysuria or increased urinary frequency.

9. I told her to call me if she felt ill.

10. We asked her to bring the following: her pain journal, her medications, and her unfilled prescriptions.

PARENTHESES

I. PROOFREADING.

1. The patient was being seen for an injured left ankle he suffered during a motorcycle accident(~~On~~ **on** a dirt race track, I believe ~~.~~). This patient has a longstanding history of depression and has expressed thoughts of suicidal ideation ~~[which~~ **(which** seemed to peak about a year ago after his girlfriend ~~died.]~~ **died).**
2. This patient is a 33-year-old female who states that she began to have problems with her balance approximately 8 years ago ~~.~~(~~her~~ **Her** complaints began after a head trauma.)Her complaints consist of fatiguing easily after prolonged activity and losing her balance during ambulation easily.(~~she~~ **She** has been a distance runner for years ~~.~~)

HYPHENS – LESSON 2

I. PROOFREADING.

1. The patient, a ~~26-year old~~ **26-year-old** female, arrived today with her ~~exhusband~~ **ex-husband** and her son.
2. On her followup, we discussed the ~~xray~~ **x-ray**, where we noted a fracture.
3. She was given an ~~anti-inflammatory~~ **anti-inflammatory** for her sprain, and we will follow up to monitor her ~~insulin dependent~~ **insulin-dependent** diabetes mellitus.
4. A ~~2-shot~~ **2-shot** T-tube cholangiogram was then performed using injections of 20 cc each of ~~one-half~~ **one-half** strength Angiovist.
5. An injection was ordered for the ~~follow-up~~ **followup** appointment.
6. There is a ~~yellow-green~~ **yellow-green** discoloration at the site of the ecchymosis that radiates 2 cm in all directions from the site.
7. This ~~12 year-old~~ **12-year-old** male presents with fatigue related to anemia.

APOSTROPHES – LESSON 1

CHALLENGE BOX.

1. **Nurse's.** Since the nurse is singular, you really don't need to think much…nearly all singular words use apostrophe s when they become possessive.
2. **Teachers'.** The word **teachers** is plural and ends in *s*, so it requires only an apostrophe.

APOSTROPHES – LESSON 2

I. MULTIPLE CHOICE.

1. men's
2. one's
3. Ross's
4. days'
5. father-in-law's
6. doctors'
7. Zenker's
8. kidneys'
9. GI's
10. x-rays
11. bone's
12. mother and father's
13. children's
14. its
15. hour's

QUOTATION MARKS

I. PROOFREADING.

1. The patient described her issue as an **"** unsteady feeling in my ~~legs~~ **legs. "**
2. ~~Stop Stop you~~ **" Stop! Stop! You** ' re trying to kill ~~me~~ **me! "** she kept screaming throughout the examination **.**
3. He described the color of the skin as **"** sea ~~green~~ **green. "**
4. When asked about the headache, she said ~~this~~ **, " This** is the worst pain I have ever ~~felt~~ **felt. "**
5. The patient repeatedly asked ~~how~~ **, " How** much will it ~~hurt~~ **hurt? "**

Capitalization

CAPITALIZATION RULES 1–5

CHALLENGE BOX.

1. She told me the feeling was "like a pinprick."
   The quote is not a complete sentence so it does not get capitalized.
2. When considering options, take several things into account: Do you want to spend a few weeks recovering now or a lifetime dealing with the pain? Do you have a means of avoiding future damage to the site? Do you have the support at home to help with recovery?
3. Of her elbow pain, she said, "The only good days I have are when I do not need to get out of bed."
4. CURRENT MEDICATIONS:
   1. Aspirin.
   2. Warfarin.

I. PROOFREADING.

1. ~~keep~~ **Keep** this in mind: ~~the~~ **The** best medicines will only work if you are taking them religiously.
2. Patient is ~~Right Hand~~ **right hand** dominant. ~~he~~ **He** has not had many blood draws in the left arm.
3. The patient was told to stick to the following diet: increased fiber, decreased dairy, and no sodas at all.
4. Some of the pain has subsided. ~~she~~ **She** says it is now 3/10.
5. ~~i~~ **I** have asked her to remain on the following medications: aspirin, beta blockers, and Lexapro.

CAPITALIZATION RULES 6-10

CHALLENGE BOX.

1. Once we get the results from Doctor Bailey, we may refer her to a pain clinic.
2. This patient suffered an injury to her femur during her work in the U.S. Postal Service.
3. This patient will be seen by Cardiology immediately and I will consult with Jared Decker, MD, FACC.
4. If we get the pulmonary tests back, we will have her follow up with East Wayne Pulmonary Center.

I. MULTIPLE CHOICE.

1. The consulting doctor ordered the patient to Radiology for an immediate x-ray.
2. At this time, we will ask the patient to follow up with Dr. Alec at the podiatry clinic.
3. He was ordered to follow a diet recommended by the American Dietetic Association.
4. The patient had been escorted to us from Early Dawn Mental Health by Officer Mason.
5. The patient presents today with an injury she received while working for the city.

CAPITALIZATION RULES 11–14

CHALLENGE BOX.
1. Tick-borne diseases like this are not uncommon in the North this time of year.
2. The patient has been exposed to severe acute respiratory syndrome, also known as SARS.
3. She is a Hispanic woman from a town east of Columbia, South Carolina.
4. If her progress continues, we will see her in July and then not again until fall.

I. TRUE/FALSE.
1. false
2. true
3. false
4. true
5. false

Agreement

TENSE AGREEMENT

I. TRUE/FALSE.
1. false
2. true
3. false
4. false
5. true
6. true
7. false
8. true
9. false
10. false

SUBJECT/VERB AGREEMENT

CHALLENGE BOX.
1. **Is** is the correct answer. **Patient** is the subject—**in addition to the parents** is an intervening phrase and cannot contain the subject.
2. **Have** is the correct answer. **Medications** is the subject closest to the verb, so the verb must agree with it.
3. **Was** is the correct answer. **Piece** is the subject—**of the fractured eyeglasses** is a prepositional phrase and cannot contain the subject.

SUBJECT/VERB AGREEMENT WITH PRONOUNS

CHALLENGE BOX.
1. **Is** is the correct answer. **Each** is the subject and is a singular pronoun—**of the pins** is a prepositional phrase and cannot contain the subject.
2. **Has** is the correct answer. **Some** is the subject. In this case it is referring to the **discomfort** (which is singular). It means part of the discomfort.
3. **Were** is the correct answer. **A number** is the subject and is plural when used this way.

REVIEW: SUBJECT/VERB AGREEMENT

I. MULTIPLE CHOICE.

1. is	2. is
3. are	4. seem
5. appears	6. is
7. were	8. appears
9. is	10. is
11. was	12. appear
13. disappears	14. is
15. seem	

PRONOUN AGREEMENT

I. MULTIPLE CHOICE.

1. their	2. it
3. their	4. its
5. its	6. it
7. it	8. it
9. it	10. they

OBJECTIVE PRONOUNS

CHALLENGE BOX.

1. **Her** is the correct answer. **Her** is the object of the preposition **with**. If you said the sentence without the words **the patient**, you would be able to choose the right pronoun easily.
2. **He** is the correct answer. The word **was** has been left off of the end of the sentence… *more enthusiastic than he was.*
3. **Whom** is the correct answer. **Whom** is the object of the preposition **from**.

POSSESSIVE PRONOUNS

I. MULTIPLE CHOICE.

1. him	2. he
3. whom	4. his
5. she	6. her
7. him	8. me
9. she	10. whom

II. FILL IN THE BLANK.

1. she	2. she
3. her	4. her
5. hers	

MODIFIER CLARITY

I. MULTIPLE CHOICE.

1. In the wounds, the sutures have been there for a week and are ready to be removed.
2. Expecting the worst, the patient was surprised to see his blood pressure was 138/78.
3. The patient was taken in a wheelchair to the examining room.
4. Describing the pain as burning and intermittent, the patient explained that the pain extends through the volar forearm.
5. After thorough counseling as to the indications, procedure, and complications of the procedure, the patient was taken to the operating room on February 4, 2006, and a splenectomy was performed.
6. After the surgery, the patient was able to walk with barely any help.
7. The patient arrived at her workplace in extreme pain.
8. Soft and nontender, the abdomen seemed no cause for concern.
9. This 50-year-old female patient with carcinoma of the left breast complains today of reflux.
10. I had seen this patient as a young child for acute appendicitis.

PARALLEL STRUCTURE

I. TRUE/FALSE.

1. true
2. false
3. false
4. true
5. false
6. false
7. true
8. true
9. false
10. false